The
Musculoskeletal
System

Penguin Library of Nursing

The Penguin Library of Nursing was
created by Penguin Education and is
published by Churchill Livingstone

The Musculoskeletal System

Orthopaedics, rheumatology and fractures

J. P. Fleetcroft MB BS, DObstRCOG, FRCS

Consultant Orthopaedic Surgeon, Medway Hospital,
Gillingham, Kent, UK; formerly Senior Surgical Officer
and Senior Registrar, Royal National Orthopaedic
Hospital, Stanmore, Middlesex, UK

CHURCHILL LIVINGSTONE

EDINBURGH LONDON MELBOURNE AND NEW YORK 1983

CHURCHILL LIVINGSTONE
Medical Division of Longman Group Limited

Distributed in the United States of America by Churchill
Livingstone Inc., 1560 Broadway, New York, N.Y. 10036, and
by associated companies, branches and representatives
throughout the world.

First published 1983

ISBN 0 443 01611 9
ISSN 0144-6592

British Library Cataloguing in Publication Data

Fleetcroft, John
    The musculoskeletal system.—(Penguin library of nursing)
    1. Musculoskeletal system
    I. Title
    617'.7   QP301

Library of Congress Cataloging in Publication Data

Fleetcroft, J. P. (John P.)
    The musculoskeletal system.
    (Penguin library of nursing)
    Bibliography: p.
    Includes index.
    1. Orthopedic nursing. 2. Orthopedia. 3. Fractures. 4.
Rheumatism. I. Title. II. Series. [DNLM: 1. Bone
diseases—Nursing texts. 2. Bone—Injury—Nursing texts. 3.
Joint diseases—Nursing texts. 4. Joints—Injury—Nursing
texts. 5. Muscular diseases—Nursing texts. WY 157.6 F594m]
    RD753.F58   1982   616.7   82-19767

Printed in Singapore by Selector Printing Co Pte Ltd

Preface

Diseases of bones and joints fall into three distinct categories—orthopaedics, traumatology and rheumatology. In this book all aspects are considered. An outline of the diseases affecting joints is arranged in two parts, one considering the generalised disorders and the other specific regional conditions. Presenting features, clinical signs, investigations, pathology and treatment (both medical and surgical) are covered. Nursing care plans are included, and details of nursing techniques will be found throughout the text, and especially in Chapter One.

This book is written for the nurse, and the presentation and content are designed to cater for the nurse embarking on training for the Orthopaedic Nursing Certificate as well as the nurse in general training. The illustrations are plentiful, providing a clear understanding of the topics considered.

I wish to thank all my colleagues who have supported me and encouraged me with the text. In particular I would like to thank the nurses who have read and criticised the text at the following hospitals: Royal National Orthopaedic Hospital, Stanmore, Edgware General Hospital, Barnet General Hospital, Watford General Hospital and the Hospital for Sick Children, Great Ormond Street, London. I am particularly indebted to my senior surgical colleagues at the same hospitals for their inspiration and training. The clear diagrams were drawn by Jane Garrud, to whom I am also most grateful. My thanks are also due to Mary Emmerson Law of Churchill Livingstone for her continued inspiration throughout the writing of this book.

London, 1983   J. P. F.

To Daphne, my wife,
in gratitude for her support throughout
the writing of this book and for her helpful criticism,
based on nursing experience

Contents

One
Basic principles

Orthopaedics

This term is derived from the Greek and is composed of two words *orthos pais*, meaning 'straight child'. Orthopaedics today is concerned with disorders of bones, joints, muscles, tendons and nerves in both adults and children. A team approach to this speciality is essential, involving representatives of all disciplines connected with the musculo-skeletal system. These include the physiotherapist, the occupational therapist, the rheumatologist, the specialist in physical medicine, the orthopaedic surgeon and the orthopaedic nurse. The radiologist provides a valuable diagnostic service which extends from the routine X-ray film or radiograph to the sophisticated arthrogram, myelogram or bone scan.

Joints, muscles, nerves and bones are the basic areas of concern for the orthopaedic nurse. To these are added the general field of trauma, which is closely associated with orthopaedics, although soft-tissue trauma to the abdomen is the province of the general surgeon and head injuries the neurosurgical speciality. There is fre-

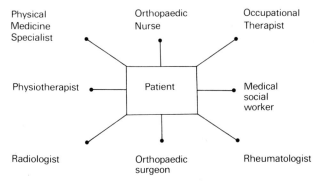

Fig. 1.1 The orthopaedic team

quently overlap between these specialities. The rheumatologist, for instance, manages the acute phases of arthritis, and the rheumatologist and the orthopaedic surgeon jointly manage chronic arthritis.

The role of the nurse is vital to the successful treatment of specific musculo-skeletal disorders and to the general wellbeing of the patient, who feels well in himself apart for the specific localised problem for which he seeks treatment. Confining a patient to bed immediately presents the problem of pressure-area care, which if neglected can lead to intractable sores which may only heal after complicated plastic surgery (see p 7). Mobilisation of joints after surgery requires both persistence and skill on the part of the nurse in conjunction with the physiotherapist.

Principles of bone growth

Bone develops in mesenchyme in the fetus, and by the sixth week of intra-uterine life a hyaline cartilage matrix consisting of cartilage cells is forming. Divisions in the cartilage denote the formation of joints, and at eight weeks gestation the strips of cartilage between the joints develop a cuff of mesenchymal cells around their centre, from which blood vessels develop and grow into the cartilage. The cells in the centre die and are replaced by primitive bone which forms the primary ossification centre. The cuff surrounding the new bone is the *periosteum*, and this cuff develops around the whole length of developing bone. Where it lies over cartilage it forms the *perichondrium*. The bone at this stage consists of a tube (the *diaphysis*) covered with periosteum, at both ends of which is a mass of cartilage (the *epiphysis*) covered with perichondrium (Fig. 1.2).

Ossification of the shafts of long bones and of the flat bones such as the pelvis, together with repair after fracture, occurs by membranous ossification. The periosteum divides into two layers, the outer the *fibrous layer*, the inner the *cambial layer*. Osteoid then separates the cambial layer from the underlying bone and cartilage. Bone salts infiltrate the osteoid. Osteocytes from the inner layer are incorporated in the mineralised osteoid (Fig. 1.3).

Bones grow from the epiphyseal growth plate by the process of enchondral ossification. In fetal life bones grow by cartilage being added to the *metaphysis*. The metaphysis is the area between the epiphyseal growth plate and the diaphysis. After birth a primary ossification centre develops in the centre of the cartilaginous epiphysis. As this develops the growth plate becomes more obvious on

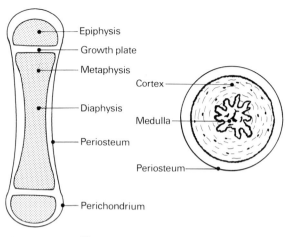

Fig. 1.2 The structure of bone

X-ray examination, as the area of translucency between the epiphysis and metaphysis. At the growth plate three zones of activity can be identified: 1. zone of cartilage growth 2. zone of cartilage transformation 3. zone of ossification.

The first layer is the zone of cartilage growth, where the chondrocytes multiply and form columns or palisades. The next zone is that of cartilage transformation, where the cells swell and accumulate water and glycogen. The cells then begin to degenerate and chondroid develops between the columns of degenerating cells. The chondroid then develops bone salts and the cells die. Blood vessels invade the areas left by the dying cells or chondrocytes. From these invading vessels bone-forming osteoblasts line the calcified chondroid, laying down osteoid in which mineral salts are deposited to form bone of the *primary spongiosa* type which fills the medullary

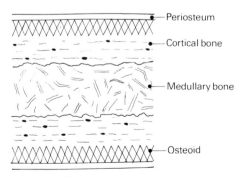

Fig. 1.3 Membranous ossification

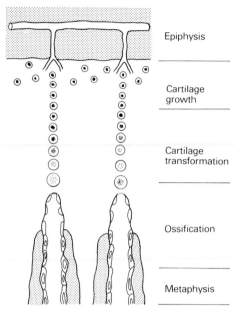

Epiphysis

Cartilage
growth

Cartilage
transformation

Ossification

Metaphysis

Fig. 1.4 Endochondral ossification

cavity of tubular bones. The primary spongiosa bone is then subsequently resorbed and replaced with more mature *trabecular bone* (Fig. 1.4).

The following are required for normal bone development: vitamin A, vitamin C, vitamin D, calcium, phosphate, growth hormone, thyroid hormone, steroids and parathormone in their correct quantities.

Growth in the length of bones occurs at the epiphyseal plate by enchondral ossification, and growth in their diameter occurs at the periosteum by membranous ossification. At the end of growth the epiphyseal plate is invaded by blood vessels and becomes ossified. Premature closure of this growth plate will cause disturbance in the growth of a bone and may cause either angulation or stunted growth in that bone.

Fracture healing

The first thing that develops around a fracture is a haematoma. Cells from the periosteum arising from the inner (cambial) layer then proliferate and form a collar of tissue around the bone ends.

Similarly, there is a proliferation of the cells in the endosteum. This cellular tissue then bridges the gap between the fractured ends of the bone, provided there is no muscle between the ends of the bone to cause an obstruction. External primary callus is thus formed. This can usually be seen on X-rays from the tenth day after the fracture. As the callus develops so the movement between the fractured bone ends reduces until the fracture becomes stable and movement ceases. The external callus is a very effective way of stabilising a fracture, and this mass of bone can be readily felt around the fracture. Structurally it is woven bone, and it is gradually removed by osteoclasts and replaced by lamellar bone, the mass of callus at the fracture being resorbed so that after remodelling has occurred there is only minimal extra bone at the fracture site.

Those surgeons who frequently fix fractures internally with plates, screws and nails (intramedullary) have shown that the amount of external callus produced at the fracture site is markedly reduced by internal fixation. That means the strength of the bone at the fracture depends solely on the method of fixation, and bone healing then occurs by bridging the fracture with lamellar bone. This occurs in the medullary cavity, and the repair is not strong enough to hold the fracture until much later than external callus, often not until about 12 months after the fracture. Hence any metal inserted across a fracture should be left untouched for at least one year before removal is contemplated.

Excessive movement at a fracture site, poor blood supply (such as in the lower third of the tibia), infection and interposed muscle will delay healing of the fracture. *Delayed union of a fracture* indicates that a fracture is taking longer to unite than predicted. If at 3 months after fracture there is no evidence of bone healing, then delayed union has occurred. If the fracture does not unite despite treatment in excess of 12 months and the X-ray shows rounding of the bone ends, *non-union* has occurred. Bone grafting of the fracture will be necessary if union is to be achieved. *Mal-union* is the term used to describe a fracture that has united with deformity at the fracture site.

Principles of diagnosis

A good history is imperative. There are no short-cuts. Patience on behalf of the doctor and nurse is essential if an accurate picture of the clinical problem is to be achieved. Listen to the patient's account of his problem. Only after this has been achieved should an examination be performed, and again this should not be confined to the local area in question. The patient must be considered in his entirety. Blood tests are invaluable; they indicate the level of calcium metabolism and hence relate to bone stock. Bone infections can be monitored by the erythrocyte sedimentation rate (ESR), and the different types of arthritis can be defined. Radiographs (X-rays) play an important role in the diagnosis of bone disorders, and the new specialised X-ray techniques—arthrography and radiculography—allow assessment of some of soft-tissue structures such as the cartilages in the knee or the intervertebral disc.

Principles of treatment

At all times the patient should be treated as a whole, and consideration of the patient's emotional needs is essential if treatment of a fracture or disease is to be successful. Orthopaedic patients are often in hospital for long periods, and neglect of the patient as a person can only lead to a breakdown in the relationship the patient has with those attending him, and prejudice the outcome of treatment.

Much of the orthopaedic surgeon's work depends on the execution of specific nursing procedures for a successful outcome. Operations on the hand require in the immediate postoperative period high elevation of the hand in a sling to prevent complications due to swelling. Hip joint replacemet demands a correct nursing technique if dislocation of the hip prothesis is to be avoided. Fractures need careful management on traction, constant attention being given to the method of traction and to any necessary adjustments. The elderly must have regular care of pressure areas if deep sores are to be prevented. Children are often in hospital for long periods and arrangements for their schooling have to be made.

Orthopaedic patients, provided that they do not have a generalised disease or infection, feel well in themselves apart from pain in a limb, and hence they can make great demands on your time.

The physiotherapist also has a very important role in the mobilisation of patients.

General nursing principles

Attention should be given to the basic nursing requirements of each patient. The elderly who are admitted with lower limb fractures often have a mild degree of heart failure with swollen ankles. They are frequently constipated, which is only aggravated by admission to hospital and traction in bed. They then feel nauseated, and stop eating a balanced diet and become dehydrated. Attention to their bowel action early will prevent the subsequent problems of impaction of faeces.

Similarly, elderly men are frequently on the verge of retention of urine and may well require catheterisation. Beware of retention of urine, as this is frequently missed until the patient is obviously uraemic.

In females the reverse applies: they are often incontinent of urine if elderly, primarily because they do not have the mobility to reach the toilet in time or are unable to summon assistance from the nursing staff. Incontinence should be managed by early catheterisation to prevent bed sores developing as the result of the patient lying in a wet bed. Catheter care is important to prevent bladder infections. Remove the catheter as soon as patient is mobile.

Communication with the patient and relatives is essential if the patient and his family are to have confidence in your nursing ability as well as the ability of the attending doctors. Give the patient time, even if you feel rushed off your feet. Make sure they understand outline of the treatment prescribed by the doctor. If you anticipate that a period of convalescence following hospital treatment is likely, alert the medical social worker early so that the necessary arrangements can be made. Enquire about the home circumstances and anticipate any help that the patient may require at home on discharge.

Pressure-area care

This is a very important part of the responsibilities of the orthopaedic nurse. Neglect of this basic care will lead to months of misery on the part of the patient and despair on the part of the nurse. The patient confined to bed, either because of treatment perscribed or because of his disability, tends to lie motionless, particularly if in pain and overweight. The body weight is therefore concentrated on the skin over the sacrum and behind the heels. Because the patient remains still, the skin over these areas becomes devoid of a blood supply (ischaemic) and then blisters. The area turns a dusky blue colour and necrosis sets in. The heels sustain a second insult. The patient is encouraged to push him- or herself up the bed by digging the heels into the bed and extending the legs. Because of their inability to move the trunk the heels lose their grip and slip down the sheet, a friction burn then occurring over the skin.

The pressure sore, if superficial, will heal in a few weeks with energetic nursing care. If loss of the skin and subcutaneous tissue is complete, then bone appears uncovered by soft tissue. The only treatment for this disaster is prolonged nursing care, and if necessary the area can be closed by a plastic surgeon. The sad fact is that if only adequate attention had been given to pressure areas from the time the patient entered the doors of the hospital, horrific pressure sores could have been be avoided.

Prolonged waiting on trolleys while the patient is transferred from one department to another is also a major contributory factor. Skin over the sacrum, heel, elbow shoulder blade and greater trochanter all requires pressure area care.

Prophylaxis

1. Turn patient regularly—2-hourly if indicated
2. Give pressure area care—soap and water, oil
3. Have the patient lying on a sheepskin
4. Apply Op-site plastic film if incontinence is a problem
5. Catheterise if incontinence of urine is a major problem
6. Use a deep foam mattress, ripple bed, low-loss air bed or water bed
7. Do not allow your patient to lie on trolleys for long periods of time
8. Encourage oral fluids and high-protein diet.

Treatment

1. Turn patient 2-hourly from side to side and use the prone position
2. Expose sore to air—use cradle
3. If the sores are very deep, deslough and pack with Eusol or similar, and repack at least twice daily
4. Various other applications include painting mercurochrome or gentian violet on the wound, and more recently Debrisan granules and Karaya powder have been advocated for application in an effort to dry the exudate from the wound. For very large sores silastic foam dressing applied as necessary may aid healing of the cavitiy.
5. It is important to take culture swabs from the sore regularly, and to maintain an adequate diet for the patient. The haemoglobin requires regular checking.

Definition of common terms

Some of the terms used to describe the movement of joints are illustrated in Figure 1.5.

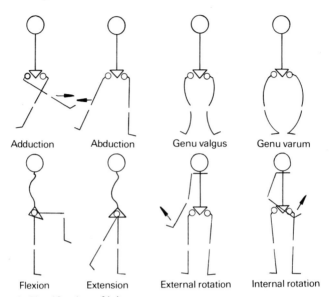

Fig. 1.5 Classification of joint movement

Abduction—the outward deviation of a limb distal to a joint
Adduction—the inward deviation of a limb distal to a joint
External rotation—the outward rotation of a bone
Internal rotation—the inward rotation of a bone
Flexion—the movement that brings bones together
Extension—the movement that takes bone apart
Supination—turning the palm to face forward
Pronation—turning the palm to face backward

Two

Generalised disorders of skeletal development

Bone may fail to be laid down correctly as a result of the following disorders:
Bone dysplasia
Metabolic disease
Endocrine disease
Abnormality in the reticulo-endothelial system
Haematological disorders
Miscellaneous conditions

Bone dysplasias

The term *dysplasia* denotes abnormal development. This abnormality may be in the epiphysis, the growth plate, the metaphysis or in the diaphysis.

Epiphyseal dysplasias

Dysplasia epiphysealis muliplex is a mild form causing little disability. The epiphyses are irregular on X-ray, affecting several joints, and there is associated stunting of the long bones (Fig. 2.1).

Dysplasia epiphysealis punctata is a more aggressive form, the epiphyses appearing stippled on X-ray.

Diastrophic dwarfism is a severe form leading to twisted feet and spine with short limbs.

Trevor's disease or dysplasia epiphysealis hemimelica affects one side of the body only. Osteochondromata develop in the epiphysis leading to progressive joint deformity.

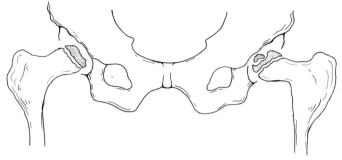

Fig. 2.1 Dysphasia epiphysealis multiplex. Note 1) the bilateral involvement of the epiphysis 2) coxa vara 3) fragmentation of the epiphysis on the left

Growth plate dysplasias

Underactivity of the growth plate leads to short bones; the end result if left uncorrected is a dwarf. The circus clown, with a relatively large head and trunk and short limbs, is the commonest example. The face has a saddle nose and frontal bossing, and there is sometimes hydrocephalus. The spinal canal is narrow and may cause symptoms of spinal stenosis in the adult. This type of dwarfing is *achondroplasia* (Fig. 2.2).

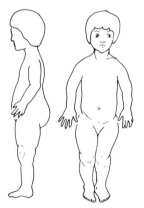

Fig. 2.2 Achondroplasia (short-limbed dwarf)

Overactivity of the growth plate results in the long bones, fingers and feet becoming excessively long. The distance from the top of the skull to the pubis is normally equal to the distance from the pubis to the sole. The arm span normally measures no more than body height. In *arachnodactyly*, or *Marfan's syndrome* the arm span and the pubis to sole measurements are increased. In addition, the fingers and toes are long and thin. This condition is associated with a high arched palate, lax joints, dislocation of the eye lenses, deafness and heart, lung and kidney disease.

Metaphyseal dysplasias

Failure of resorption of primitive bone to allow new bone to be produced in the mature form, with cancellous bone and cortical bone, results in there being no medullary cavity, the bone becoming virtually solid, like marble. Albers-Schönberg first described this condition which is known as *osteopetrosis* (Fig. 2.3). The severe form is noticed at birth, Anaemia, cranial nerve palsies and dwarfing are typical. A milder form exists, osteopetrosis tarda, and fragile bones developing pathological fractures associated with anaemia are characteristic of this.

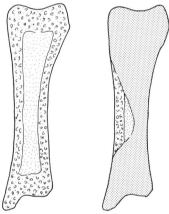

Fig. 2.3 Left: normal bone Right: osteopetrosis (marble bone)

Diaphyseal dysplasias

Osteogenesis imperfecta is an example of a dysplasia affecting the diaphysis. Primitive bone is laid down normally, but the collagen is abnormal and unable to mature, preventing the formation of normal compact bone. The bones are fragile and deform and fracture easily. The abnormality in collagen may cause blue sclera in the eyes, thin skin, poor teeth, lax joints and macular bleeding in the eye.

The mild form may only be noticed in the older child who has repeated fractures of the limbs without significant trauma. The sclera will be blue and a family history is likely. The fractures are man-

aged in a routine manner and the patient is little disabled. The severe form presents a challenge to the patient as to those caring for
him. The bones are very fragile, frequently fractured at birth. Deformity is common, with bowing of the long bones. The spine may
develop a curvature. Management of the fractures is difficult, the
bones often requiring intramedullary nailing to correct deformity at
the fracture site. The bones frequently bow, and multiple osteotomies are performed to correct alignment. Respiratory insufficiency
may threaten life in the infant. Because the bones are so fragile,
careful handling of the patient is essential, particularly when splints
are in use. Fractures may occur if the splint is allowed to hang unsupported, digging into the limb. Children suffering from
osteogenesis imperfecta are of normal intellligence and frequently
become frustrated with their plight (Fig. 2.4).

Metabolic disorders

Rickets and osteomalacia

Rickets and osteomalacia are the same condition, rickets affecting
children and osteomalacia affecting adults. Bone fails to be suf-
ficiently mineralised with calcium and phosphate. Vitamin D is
responsible for the deposition of calcium in bone as well as its
absorption from the small intestine (Fig. 2.5).

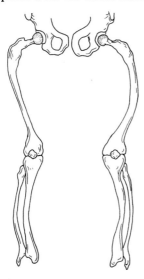

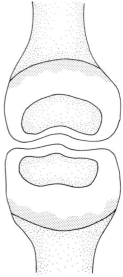

Fig. 2.4 Osteogenesis imperfecta
(fragile bone disease)

Fig. 2.5 Rickets. Note 1) wide
epiphyseal plate 2) cupping of
metaphysis

Nutritional rickets

This condition is due to a deficiency in vitamin D, either due to
dietary lack—vitamin D is found in eggs, fish liver oil, butter, mar-
garine—or due to lack of exposure to sunlight, which converts its
precursor in the skin into Vitamin D. Failure of absorption of fats
from the small intestine, as is found in coelia disease and fibro-
cystic disease of the pancreas, will also reduce the absorption of
vitamin D. Nutritional rickets commonly presents around the
second year of life with bowing of the legs, swollen wrists and
prominent costochondral junctions (rickety rosary) and failure to
thrive. The skull is enlarged, with a large fontanelle giving the
appearance of a 'hot cross bun'. Walking is achieved late and the
muscles are poorly developed.

X-rays reveal wide epiphyseal plates and wide metaphyses with
cupping. The serum calcium is normal or slightly lowered, the
serum phosphate is low and the alkaline phosphatase is raised.
Daily vitamin D2 (calciferol) 1500 to 5000 units will restore the
calcium metabolism to normal within four weeks.

Vitamin D with calcium supplements is given for as long as
necessary to establish a well-balanced diet, and growth returns to
normal. Bowing of the legs may require osteotomy to correct the
deformity.

Renal osteodystrophy

This affects older children and is due to impaired renal function.
Phosphates are not excreted, causing the serum phosphate level to
rise. This in turn causes a drop in the level of serum calcium,
which stimulates the parathyroids to secrete parathormone to raise
the serum calcium. Hence the changes are a mixture of rickets and
hyperparathyroidism. The appearance at X-ray is characteristic.
Treatment is directed towards restoring kidney function.

Vitamin D-resistant rickets.

In this group the patient does not respond to normal doses of
vitamin D but does respond to high doses. One type, *phosphaturic
rickets*, is caused by an excessive output of phosphates in the urine.
The patient will require to take high doses of vitamin D all his life,
about 100 000 units daily. There is a danger of hypercalcaemia
which, should it occur, can be controlled with cortisone. Ideally, if
elective surgery is planned, vitamin D should be withheld six weeks
prior to and six weeks after operation.

Another variant is caused by failure of the kidney tubule to re-sorb bicarbonate. This causes the urine to be alkaline, and calcium is lost in high quantities. This is known as *renal tubular acidosis*.

Fanconi syndrome

This is the result of multiple tubular defects within the kidney. Its characteristics are dwarfism, rickets, albuminuria, aminoaciduria, renal glycosuria, low serum phosphate and high blood urea. Treatment of the rickets is undertaken in close collaboration with the paediatrician, and frequently control of renal function reverses the bone changes without requiring the administration of vitamin D.

Correction of deformity in rickets

After the institution of medical treatment, correction of bowing of the femur or tibia, or both, may be considered. Minor deformity may correct with bone growth and moulding, but major bowing re-quires surgical correction by osteotomy-osteoclasis. The bone is cut across leaving the periosteum on one side intact, correction of de-formity being achieved by hinging the bone on the intact perios-teum. The correction is maintained in plaster of Paris until sound union has occured at the osteotomy site, which usually happens within six weeks.

Osteomalacia

This is rare except in certain Asiatic lands, although in the UK it may occur in elderly ladies. It is the adult counterpart of the nutri-tional rickets seen in children. Osteomalacia in adults presents with fractures rather than deformity and the X-ray appearances are char-acteristic. Spontaneous fractures are seen, usually affecting only one cortex and painless, in the pelvic and long bones. These are called *Looser's zones*. The blood biochemistry is the same as for nu-tritional rickets. Treatment is to give vitamin D.

Scurvy

Deficiency of vitamin C (ascorbic acid) is associated with haemor-rhage from the gums, beneath the periosteum, causing the limb to become painful and swollen (the child therefore not using it), and around the eye, although haemorrhage may occur anywhere. The child is usually between 6 and 12 months old, is irritable and fails to thrive. Vitamin C is found in fresh milk and orange juice, but is inactivated by boiling. Scurvy is rare today, but may occur in a baby fed on boiled milk and orange juice that has also been boiled.

The pain of a subperiosteal bleed may cause a pseudoparalysis. The periosteum is raised by the haemorrhage and new bone is formed underneath, causing the bone to be grossly thickened. The metaphysis may lose its density and on X-ray gives the appearance of ground glass.

Vitamin C is given in the established case, 100 mg to 200 mg daily, and attention is given to diet. In severe cases bed rest may be necessary.

Scurvy may also affect adults; the skin may fail to heal after minor cuts and haemorrhages under the skin may occur. Bone is not affected as it is in the child.

Endocrine disorders

Parathyroid

There are four parathyroid glands situated on the posterior aspect of the thyroid gland. Overactivity of one of these glands, caused by an adenoma, produces an excess of parathormone. Excessive parathormone mobilises calcium from bone, raising the serum level. Cysts develop in bone and the bones soften. The patient, an adult, is weak and complains of bone pain. *Von Recklinghausen's disease, generalised osteitis fibrosa cystica* and *hyperparathyroidism* are all titles that describe this parathyroid osteodystrophy. Treatment is directed at locating the adenoma and removing it.

Thyroid

Cretinism is a congenital deficiency of thyroid hormone secretion. If the child remains untreated growth becomes stunted, the hands are broad and fingers short, the anterior fontanelle remains open, the neck is short and thick and there is a slit appearance to the eyes with a protruding tongue. Mental retardation occurs and the milestones in development are delayed. The epiphyses may become irregular, appearing on X-ray like Perthes' disease. The first two lumbar vertebrae also have a characteristic appearance.

Pituitary

Overproduction of growth hormone in childhood leads to *gigantism,* due to skeletal overgrowth. The child may grow to a height of seven feet if untreated.

In adults the growth plates are closed so the length of the bone cannot increase. The bones however can increase in thickness and this is particularly true of the hands and feet, skull and mandible which all enlarge. This is called *acromegaly*.

Adrenal

Oversecretion of hydrocortisone produces osteoporosis, and the bones fracture without severe force. Cushing's syndrome is the commonest cause.

Disorders of the reticulo-endothelial system

This group encompasses those conditions where deposits of granulomatous tissue occur in bone or elsewhere. They mostly affect children or young adults.

Hand-Schüller-Christian disease

Fibrosis is a feature of the deposits in this condition. Histiocytes accumulate lipoid in bone and rupture; then fibrosis occurs. The lesions appear as punched-out holes on X-ray. If the pituitary becomes involved, diabetes insipidus occurs.

Eosinophilic granuloma

This presents as a solitary bone lesion, frequently in a vertebral body, appearing like a solitary bone cyst. The lesion contains an infiltration of eosinophils within a mass of histiocytes. The lesion frequently resolves spontaneously to a normal appearance (Fig. 2.6).

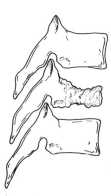

Fig. 2.6 Eosinophilic granuloma of vertebral body of the spine

Letterer-Siwe disease

This is a more widespread form of the Hand-Schüller-Christian type of disease, with the spleen, liver and lymph nodes also involved. The patient looks pale and develops a bleeding disorder.

Gaucher's disease

The infiltration in this type is of histiocytes containing a lipoid cerebroside called kerasin. Diagnosis is confirmed by sternal marrow biopsy.

Niemann-Pick disease

This is similar to Gaucher's disease. It almost always fatal, the lipoid in the cells being one of the phosphosphingosides.

Haematological disorders

Sickle cell anaemia

This is a disease of blood corpuscles affecting negroes and to a lesser extent Jamaicans. The affected corpuscle contains Haemaglobin S. If only one gene is Hbs then the disease is called *trait*, and the patient is a carrier. If two genes are abnormal then sickle cell anaemia occurs. This is characterised by crises where the abnormal corpuscles haemolyse and the debris blocks the capillaries. Bone becomes infarcted, causing pain, and the affected bone may later sequestrate, associated with a secondary periostitis.

Haemorrhagic disorders

Where there is a lack of one of the clotting factors in the blood as in *haemophilia* (factor VIII) or *Christmas disease* (factor IX), or where there is an abnormality in the walls of the capillaries as in *von Willebrand's disease*, haemorrhage as the result of minor trauma fails to stop and large haematomata result. These may be subcutaneous, within the muscle, around nerves or in a joint. As well as a fall in the circulating blood volume, local damage occurs to the tissue within the haemorrhage. Muscles become ischaemic and fibrose, developing a contracture. The nerves may be compressed, causing paresis and paralysis in the area supplied by the nerve, and haemorrhage into joints leads to avascular necrosis of the epiphysis, resulting in joint destruction. Subperiosteal haemorrhages occur and these eventually form a bone cyst.

Treatment is directed at arresting the bleeding by giving the appropriate blood factor, and local measures involve splintage of the affected area.

Miscellaneous conditions

Ehlers-Danlos syndrome

This syndrome is the result of an abnormality in collagen and therefore affects skin, muscle and ligaments. The skin is very supple and can be readily stretched, the joints are lax and can be put through an abnormal range of movement. Scoliosis may also be present. Congenital dislocation of the hip and club foot (congenital talipes equinovarus, CTEV) are frequently present.

Arthrogryposis multiplex congenita

Joints have a limited range of movement, the muscles are often hypoplastic and soft tissue webbing across joints is often present. This condition is present at birth and is non-progressive. These affected are frequently highly intelligent. Treatment is directed toward achieving joint movement and functional mobility. Dislocation of the hips and club foot may also required treatment. The Freeman-Sheldon syndrome, otherwise known as the whistling face syndrome, may appear similar to AMC but the facial features are distinctive.

Neurofibromatosis

Von Recklinghausen, in 1882, demonstrated the presence of nerves in fibromata characteristic of this condition. The skin contains many nodules (*neurofibromata*) and the skin has areas of pigment (*café-au-lait spots*). Neurofibromata are found along the nerves, and in the peripheral nerves may be seen and felt. Neurofibromata of the spinal nerves may become dumb-bell shaped, causing a pressure erosion of the surrounding bone. Scoliosis is common in more than 25 per cent of cases and overgrowth of a limb is common. Pseudarthrosis of the tibia may occur, due to a neurofibroma pres-

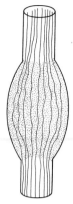

Fig. 2.7 Neurofibromatosis. Neurofibroma in the nerve

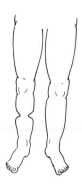

Fig. 2.8 Congenital constriction ring

ent in the bone. Sarcomatous change in the neurofiromata has been known to occur (Fig. 2.7).

Constriction rings

These are rings encircling limbs either below the elbow or below the knee. They may be simple ring constrictions of skin and sub-cutaneous tissue or associated with lymphoedema and limb deformity. The rings can be released and lengthened by Z-plasty (Fig. 2.8).

Summary of the generalised bone disorders

1. Bone dysplasias

Dysplasia epiphysealis multiplex—abnormal epiphyses
Achondroplasia—dwarf, circus clown
Marfan's syndrome—arachnoidactyly
Osteopetrosis—marble bones
Osteogenesis imperfecta—fragile bones

2. Metabolic disorders

Rickets—vitamin D deficiency
Osteomalacia—adult form of ricketts
Scurvy—vitamin C deficiency

3. Endocrine disorders

Hyperparathyroidism—overactive parathyroid
Cretinism—underactive thyroid
Acromegaly—excess of growth hormone
Cushing's syndrome—excess of hydrocortisone

4. Reticulo-endothelial disorders

Hand-Schüller-Christian disease—widespread fibrosis occurs
Eosinophilic granuloma—solitary bone lesion
Letter-Siwe disease—bleeding disorder—severe form of Hand-Schüller-Christian disease
Gaucher's disease—lipoid storage disease (kerasin)
Niemann-Pick disease—lipoid storage disease (phosphosphingosides)

5. Haematological disorders

Sickle cell anaemia—Hbs
Haemophilia—factor VIII deficiency
Christmas disease—factor IX deficiency
Von Willebrand's disease—blood vessel disorder ·

6. Miscellaneous conditions

Ehlers-Danlos syndrome—lax joints
Arthrogryposis—stiff joints
Neurofibromatosis—fibromata in nerves
Constriction rings

Three

Arthritis and rheumatic diseases

This chapter deals with those types of arthritis that are not due to a specific pyogenic infection. The arthritis may be the result of destruction of the joint by an inflammatory process within the lining of the joint (the *synovium*) as in *rheumatoid arthritis*, or the arthritis may develop as a result in the failure of the articular cartilage repair as in *osteoarthritis*.

Pain in muscles around the shoulder and back is often referred to as *fibrositis* or *muscular rheumatism*. It has been well established that these tender areas are the result of nerve root irritation around the exit foramina of the nerve root from the spine by a prolapsed disc, or hypertrophy of the posterior facet joints in the spine. Treatment of the respective areas in the spine brings relief of the symptoms.

The general features of the different types of arthritis will be discussed, but details of treatment for individual joints should be sought in the respective chapters. Arthritis caused by specific pyogenic infections (*septic arthritis*) is discussed with other infections of bone in Chapter Four.

Osteoarthritis

This is a very different condition from rheumatoid arthritis. Instead of the joint surface being destroyed by an inflammatory disease, it fails to retain its integrity because the normal healing of articular cartilage is inadequate, leaving damaged areas within the joint unrepaired. These create an uneven surface and cause further damage to the joint surface. Failure of the normal healing of articular cartilage is related to aging.

Predisposing factors to the development of osteoarthritis are:

1. Incongruity of joint surface, such as a previous fracture affecting the joint surface (Fig. 3.1(2))

2. Instability of the joint, as in congenital dislocation of the hip
3. Avascular necrosis, as in Perthes' disease (Fig. 3.1(3))
4. Increased areas of weight loading due to deformity, as in coxa vara of the hip
5. Direct injury (Fig. 3.1(4))
6. Generalised diseases, such as hypothyroidism
7. Idiopathic (unknown)

If a single joint is affected, then a specific cause for the arthritis may be obvious, but there is another variety of the arthritis that affects several joints, usually symmetrically. Often the distal joints of the fingers become enlarged, forming Herberden's nodes. The elderly are affected by this type.

Osteoarthritis presents with pain in the affected joint. The pain may lead to muscle spasm and deformity. Joint movement is reduced and if the lower limb is affected walking becomes progressively more painful. Pain is initially related to movement, but as the arthritis develops pain occurs at rest and then at night.

Treatment initially is with local methods: rest, gentle heat, analgesics. The physiotherapist may apply traction with benefit, and gently exercise the joint. Heat can be applied by massage of the area round the joint, short wave diathermy or infra-red light. More recent developments have been the use of ultrasound. Combined with these specific treatments, loss of excess body weight is essential, and suitable dieting important.

After these methods have been tried, residual pain may respond to one of the many anti-inflammatory drugs now available. Indomethacin (Indocid) and butazolidine were amongst the earlier preparations, but care must be taken with these drugs as they may cause gastric ulceration. Some of the newer preparations claim not to have this side-effect, but they may not be quite as potent as the earlier drugs. Aspirin has anti-inflammatory properties as well as an analgesic effect.

Surgery to an arthritic joint is only considered when these above measures have been tried and failed to relieve pain. Many patients with grossly arthritic joints gain pain relief with local treatment measures, regain sufficient mobility for their requirements, and never require joint surgery.

Wherever possible, surgery is directed at realigning the joint so that parts of the articular cartilage that remain are so placed that they bear the maximum weight-load passing through the joint. Hence in the hip an osteotomy of the proximal femur in the subtrochanteric region will allow the hip to be placed in an optimum

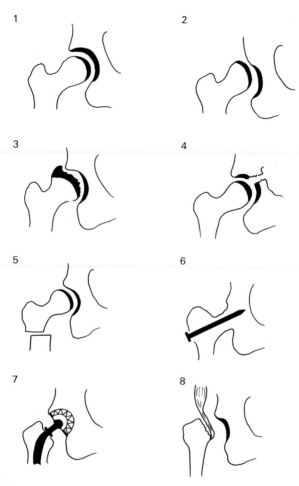

Fig. 3.1 The arthritic hip: 1) normal hip 2) lack of congruity between the two parts of the joint 3) avascular necrosis 4) fracture and dislocation of the hip joint, predisposing to arthritis 5) osteotomy 6) arthrodesis 7) total hip replacement 8) excision arthroplasty (Girdlestone's—see also Chapter Eleven)

position after careful radiographic study of the joint. *McMurray osteotomy* involves medial displacement of the distal femoral shaft, a *valgus* osteotomy increases the neck-shaft angle, and a *varus osteotomy* decreases this angle. The McMurray is fixed with a spline and the other two with a nail and plate. After this procedure pain relief may be sustained for over 10 years (Fig. 3.1(5)).

Only after this kind of surgery has been considered should joint replacement be entertained. Joint replacements are very successful

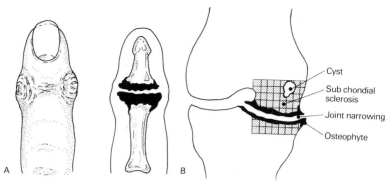

Fig. 3.2 Osteoarthritis—features appearing at X-ray. A) osteoarthritis of the finger, showing Herberdens nodes B) sclerosis of bone associated with cyst formation

in the short-term, but a significant number still require reoperation because of infection, loosening or breakage. Reoperation is not easy, and if the implant fails amputation may be the only alternative (Fig. 3.1(7)).

In the younger patient arthrodesis (fusion) of the affected joint may be appropriate provided that only one joint is involved (Fig. 3.1(6)).

The X-ray features of osteoarthritis (see Fig. 3.2) are:

   1. Narrowing of joint surface
   2. Sclerosis of bone adjacent to joint with cyst formation
   3. Osteophyte formation, new bone formation at periphery of joint

Rheumatoid arthritis

This is a systemic disease affecting joints, tendons, skin and blood vessels. It affects both adults and children, and the disease may vary considerably in its presentation, duration and extent of joint involvement. Rheumatoid arthritis tends to 'burn out' after several years, and osteoarthritis becomes superimposed on the changes already produced by the rheumatoid arthritis. The disease in children is described under the separate heading of Juvenile Rheumatoid Arthritis.

The disease affects a younger age group than osteoarthritis, and the onset is an insiduous symmetrical polyarthritis. The smaller joints are affected initially, i.e. fingers, toes, wrists and neck, but later spread to the knees and hips may occur. The cause of the disease is as yet unknown. Progressive inflammation of the synovium lining joints and tendon sheaths causes synovial thickening, and the characteristic *pannus* forms. This consists of chronic granulation tissue, which produces enzymes that destroy joint articular cartilage, causing joint destruction. The pannus from a joint may cause local pressure on neighbouring tendons, causing them to rupture. This commonly occurs with the extensor tendons at the wrist. Should the arthritis persist despite all efforts at treatment, the joint becomes totally destroyed and a bony ankylosis occurs. Fingers and toes dislocate at the metacarpo- or metatarso-phalangeal joints due to destruction of the joint ligaments and capsule, and in the hand the characteristic rheumatoid deformity develops with the fingers subluxating to the ulnar side (Fig. 3.3a). Rheumatoid nodules are found in the skin, particularly over pressure areas such as the elbow or buttock (Fig. 3.3b). The blood vessels may also be affected, a vasculitis developing, usually involving the smaller vessels. A peripheral neuropathy may also present in rheumatoid arthritis, a mild sensory loss with absent ankle jerks being the commonest presentation. Compression of the median nerve as it passes through the carpal tunnel—*carpal tunnel syndrome*—may also develop. The lungs may be affected, with the onset of a pleural effusion, and keratoconjunctivitis occurs in the eyes in rheumatoid arthritis. It should be noted that in the sero-negative arthritides an iridocyclitis develops (see Juvenile Rheumatoid Arthritis). Anaemia of the iron deficiency type may occur.

Rheumatoid arthritis in adults is usually seropositive, that is, the blood contains *rheumatoid factor*, which is an abnormal globulin (IgM). This globulin can be detected by the Latex R. A. Fixation Test or the Rose-Waaler sheep-cell agglutination test. The ESR (erythrocyte sedimentation rate) is raised and a mild anaemia is common.

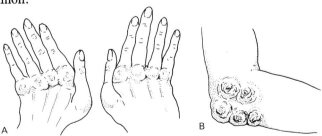

A   B

Fig. 3.3 Features of rheumatoid arthritis. A) Rheumatoid arthritis of the hands, showing characteristic deformity B) Rheumatoid nodules of the elbow

Radiological features of rheumatoid arthritis in the early stages are difficult to find. There may be some osteoporosis; later erosions occur and then the joint space becomes narrowed. Later still subchondral sclerosis develops, together with cyst formation. Osteoarthritis may be superimposed over the rheumatoid changes when the disease has burnt out. Radiographs of the hands and feet are useful in the early diagnosis of rheumatoid arthritis, being studied particularly for evidence of erosions.

Although rheumatoid arthritis commences as a generalised illness, with malaise, weight loss and tiredness, it is not until swelling of several joints simultaneously is noticed that the diagnosis is suspected. Joint pains then develop with increasing swelling and stiffness of the joints. In the initial stages of the disease rest is important, and if necessary this should be in hospital. After the instigation of anti-inflammatory drugs and a response in the way of reduced swelling and stiffness, mobilisation is then commenced. Surgery plays a part in the early stage of the disease if synovial swelling does not respond to medication, a synovectomy being performed.

The salicylates were the first line of treatment until fairly recently, but they have been superseded by the new non-steroidal anti-inflammatory drugs. These include the propionic acid derivatives ibuprofen (Brufen), naproxen (Naprosyn) and fenoprofen (Fenopron), the fenamates alclofenac (Prinalgin) and fenclofenac (Flenac), phenylbutazone and indomethacin. Should these be ineffective, gold can be given intramuscularly as sodium aurthiomalate. Care must be taken to monitor the patient and report any skin rash or tendency to haemorrhage, and repeated blood sampling is required as the white cell count may fall. Systemic steroids may be used, but these are accompanied by well-established side-effects, while the use of adrenocorticotropic hormone (ACTH) may produce the same effect without the side-effects. More recently, some physicians have been giving immunosuppressive drugs.

Surgery in rheumatoid arthritis may be directed at preventing deformity by excising the inflamed synovium (synovectomy) in the early stages of the disease, and this is valuable in the fingers and knees where ligament and tendon rupture may be prevented. Otherwise, surgery is aimed at restoring joint function by correcting deformity, such as valgus and varus knee deformity, or at relieving pain by replacing the affected joint with an artificial joint (such as in the hip or knee), by fusing the affected joint (usually only applicable to the small joints of the hand or an unstable neck) or by performing an excision arthroplasty (commonly performed as Fow-

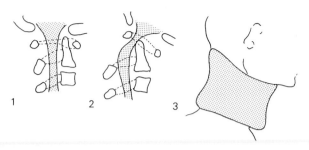

Fig. 3.4 Instability of the cervical spine in rheumatoid arthritis 1) extension 2) flexion, with compression of the spinal cord 3) stabilisation in a cervical collar

ler's operation, on the feet), where the joint is excised allowing movement.

Specific operations in rheumatoid arthritis

Neck. Instability between the first and second cervical vertebrae may occur due to destruction of the odontoid peg by the disease. Fusion of these two vertebrae posteriorly is a very satisfactory method of stabilisation (Fig. 3.4). It is worth noting that in up to 10 per cent of all patients with rheumatoid have instability at this level, and that it is therefore important to X-ray this region before any anaesthetic is administered.

Hands and Wrists. Destruction of the metacarpophalangeal joints allows the fingers to sublux towards the ulnar side. Tendon function is then impaired and finger function lost. Replacement of these joints and silastic spacers (Swanson) restores function (Fig. 3.5). Tendon rupture is common on the back of the wrist involving the extensor tendons. The tendons are repaired with excision of inflamed synovium and the distal end of the ulna. Fusion of the wrist joint will provide a stable hand if the carpus has been severely affected.

Hips. Replacement of the rheumatoid hip with a total hip replacement both relieves pain and restores function, the latter being appreciated if the knees and feet are also affected.

Knees. As mentionned above, synovectomy of the knee in the early stages of the disease may prevent serious destruction of the knee developing later. Should deformity have developed, osteotomy to

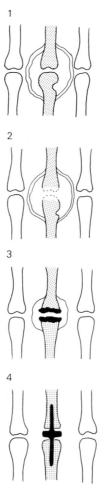

Fig. 3.5 The progress of rheumatoid arthritis of the fingers. 1) early stage of the disease, with synovial thickening and erosion 2) destruction of articular cartilage 3) late rheumatoid arthritis with secondary osteoarthritis 4) silastic spacer in finger joint

correct the deformity, either upper tibial or supracondylar in the femur or the Benjamin osteotomy may relieve pain and restore function. Should the joint be severely affected, joint replacement may be indicated. Arthrodesis of the knee is only indicated if the hip above is not severely affected.

Feet. Destruction of the metatarsophalangeal joints produces a painful foot with prominent metatarsal heads and overlying callosities. Excision of the metatarsal heads of all the toes (Fowler's operation) produces a foot that will fit a normal shoe and is no longer painful.

Mobilisation of the severely affected patient

The skilled services of the physiotherapist and occupational therapist can transform the life of a severely handicapped rheumatoid. The design of splints made from the modern heat-malleable plastics, materials to aid eating and writing and the adaptation of taps and other fittings in the home so that they can be operated can restore a certain degree of independence for the patient.

Juvenile rheumatoid arthritis

Rheumatoid occurring in children sixteen years and under falls in this group. There is a peak of incidence between one and three years of age and a further peak around puberty.

1. Still's disease

This is the systemic type described by Still in 1897. He noted that, in addition to joint involvement, there was splenomegaly, hepatomegaly and lymphadenopathy. The child had a fever, high in the evening and normal in the morning. Still's disease is usually polyarticular but may be pauciarticular, and is sometimes accompanied by a maculopapular rash for a few days. Chronic iridocyclitis may develop and this may lead to permanent ocular damage. Children between 1 and 5 years are found in this group, with an equal sex incidence.

2. Polyarticular rheumatoid arthritis

This is by far the commonest group, where systemic disease is not prominent. The knees, hands and feet are involved. Disease in the apophysial joints of the cervical spine may cause a torticollis to develop and subluxation of the second cervical vertebra on the third may occur. Similarly, disease in the transverse ligament between the odontoid process of the second cervical vertebra (the axis) and the arch of the first cervical vertebra (the atlas) may cause dislocation at this level with potential danger to the spinal cord. In older children with this type, elbow nodules develop and they are seropositive with a predominance of girls.

3. Pauciarticular rheumatoid arthritis

In this group four or less joints are involved.

Treatment

The same principles apply as for the treatment of the adult form of the disease, although care must be taken not to arrest growth, particularly when using steroids. Children with Still's disease, the systemic type in the younger child, are especially at risk because of the amount of growth still to occur. Stunting of growth and osteoporosis, if they develop, compound the disability caused by the disease itself, and stress fractures may occur.

Destruction of major joints such as the hip may be so advanced as to merit total hip replacement, with a prosthesis designed with a narrow stem suitable for a narrow femoral shaft.

Ankylosing spondilitis

If untreated this disease causes the whole length of the spine to become solid by ossification of the ligaments and joints, the patient adopting the characteristic posture of a grossly rounded back with the face pointing to the floor (Fig. 3.6). More frequent in men, this disease starts between the age of fifteen and thirty-five. There is a

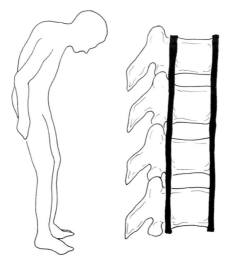

Fig. 3.6 Ankylosing spondylitis. Note the calcification of the anterior longitudinal ligament, forming 'bamboo spine'

familial tendency. The eye may become involved developing an iridiocyclitis.

Early morning spinal stiffness with low back pain is the commonest form of presentation, and there may be tenderness in the heels or sterno-manubrial joint. Chest expansion is limited to less than 5 cm and spinal movements are also limited. The ESR is raised, and frequently the serum contains an abnormal antigen, HL-A B27.

X-rays are diagnostic showing obliteration of the sacro-iliac joints and ossification in the anterior longitudinal ligament of the spine, forming the 'bamboo' spine (Fig. 3.6).

Treatment has changed over the past decades. Originally radiotherapy was given, but this was associated with subsequent malignant disease. The present treatment involves early mobilisation of the spine in a physiotherapy department with the administration of anti-inflammatory drugs.

Crystalline arthritis

In this group crystals appear in the joint and cause inflammation. Two varieties occur, gout and pseudogout.

In gout the crystals involved are of uric acid. The blood levels of uric acid are raised. The commonest joint to be affected is the metatarso-phalangeal joint of the great toe (hallux). Deposits of uric acid are sometimes found in the cartilage of the eyelid, nose and ears. Uric acid stones may also develop in the renal tract. The diagnosis is made by examining a sample of joint fluid and estimating the the blood uric acid level.

Pseudogout is very similar to gout, but the crystal that is deposited in the joint is calcium pyrophosphate. The distinction is made by finding a normal uric acid level in the blood, and by polarised light microscopy of the joint fluid.

Treatment of gout is with probenecid to reduce the level of uric acid in the blood. Pseudogout is treated with anti-inflammatory drugs alone.

Neuropathic joints

If a joint loses its sensory nerve supply, pain is not appreciated. Hence there is no restraining influence on the joint, and it will be loaded far beyond what it should carry. This in turn prevents the normal continuous process of healing of the joint cartilage. The result is continuous destruction of the joint, which is, however, free of pain. The causes of such a loss of nerve supply are: 1. Infective —syphilis 2. Diabetic 3. Failure of nerve development—spina bifida 4. Spinal cord disease.

Joints thus affected are also known as *Charcot joints* after Charcot, who described them as a feature of syphilis.

Four

Bone infections

Infections in bone occur either by spread from the blood stream
—*haematogenous osteomyelitis*—or by contamination from the skin
and environment, as in compound fractures. The infection may be
acute, subacute or *chronic*. A joint also may be infected by organisms
circulating in the blood stream, causing *septic arthritis*.

Osteomyelitis

Acute osteomyelitis

This is an important disease of childhood and also affects adults.
The organism may arise from a septic focus anywhere in the body.
The infection reaches bone through the bloodstream and the organism lodges in the metaphysis, where the infection becomes established. General malaise develops, with pain around the joint
adjacent to the metaphysis. If the lower limb is affected the child
may limp or refuse to walk.

The untreated infection will cause the child to become toxic,
with a pyrexia. The skin around the infected bone becomes red and
an abscess later develops. The infected bone develops an abscess
which penetrates through the cortex, at first raising the periosteum
then breaking through to the subcutaneous tissue then through the
skin. This sequence of events is very rarely seen today because of
the advent of antibiotics and surgical drainage of the infection in
the early phase of the disease.

Chronic infection then becomes established within the bone, the
thickened periosteum ossifying and producing an involucrum and
dead pieces of bone—*sequestrum*—being periodically discharged
from the wound. Once chronic infection is established clearance of
the infection is virtually impossible (Fig. 4.1).

The commonest organism found in acute osteomyelitis is *Staphylococcus*, and *Streptococcus, Pneumococcus, Proteus* and *Salmonella* are

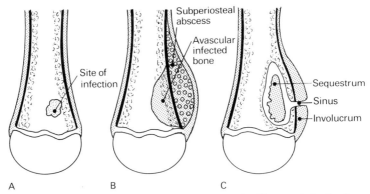

Fig. 4.1 The progress of infection in osteomyelitis. A) acute infection in the metaphysis B) pus has escaped through the cortex to form a subperiosteal abscess C) an avascular segment has separated as sequestrum and a sinus has become established through which pus escapes

also found in this condition. The infection commences in the most vascular part of the bone, the metaphysis, and in children does not penetrate the cartilage of the epiphyseal plate. The joint is therefore only affected if the metaphysis is included within the joint, and this is possible only if the capsule is attached on the metaphyseal bone. In these cases only, a septic arthritis develops, and is therefore secondary to the primary infection in the metaphysis. The hip is particularly prone to a secondary septic arthritis.

Treatment of acute osteomyelitis is a little controversial, as two schools of thought exist. The long-established treatment has been wide surgical drainage, but since the advent of antibiotics one school feels that antibiotics alone are sufficient, whereas the other school combines a limited surgical approach with the administration of antibiotics as soon as a specimen of pus has been obtained. Most surgeons favour the second method, because if antibiotic treatment alone does not completely eradicate the infection, chronic infection will become established—which would be a tragedy. As soon as the diagnosis is confirmed, the child is admitted to hospital. A search is made for the site of a nidus of infection which may have given rise to a bacteraemia. Blood samples are taken for a full blood count, ESR, blood culture and antibody titres. X-rays of the affected bone do not show any changes for at least 10 days. The child is prepared for the operating theatre.

The surgeon will drill some holes in the metaphysis, to reduce the pressure within the medullary cavity of the bone, and will take swabs of any pus that is found. The wound is closed and antibiotics can be given now that a swab has been taken and culture of the pus has begun. After 48 hours the culture is read and any necessary changes are made to the antibiotic regime. The patient is kept in bed until the wound has healed. Antibiotics should be continued for 3 months to prevent the infection becoming chronic.

Complications associated with ineffective treatment of acute osteomyelitis are:

1. Septicaemia
2. Septic arthritis of a neighbouring joint
3. Damage to the growth plate causing growth retardation
4. Chronic osteomyelitis

Subacute osteomyelitis (Brodie's abscess)

A localised abscess forming in adult bone with an insidious onset is characteristic of this form of osteomyelitis. On the X-ray film there is a well circumscribed lesion in the bone. Treatment is surgical; the cortical bone overlying the abscess is opened and the cavity curetted. Antibiotics are given after culture of the abscess and continued for 3 months (Fig. 4.2).

Chronic osteomyelitis

This inevitably follows acute osteomyelitis which has not been totally eradicated. The chronic infection presents as recurring pain in the affected limb with discharging sinuses from time to time. Frequently an involucrum develops (Fig. 4.3) and sequestra discharge from the wound periodically. A long-term course of antibiotics may suppress the infection. Sequestra and a chronic

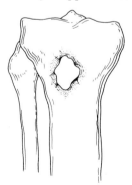

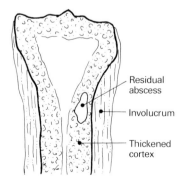

Residual abscess

Involucrum

Thickened cortex

Fig. 4.2 Brodie's abscess. Cavity in bone surrounded by ring of sclerotic bone.

Fig. 4.3 Chronic osteomyelitis

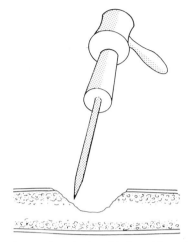

Fig. 4.4 Method of removing dead and infected bone in chronic osteomyelitis

discharging sinus require surgical exploration. A gutter is cut in the bone and sequestra are removed with chronically infected medullary bone. Recently, a chain of beads containing antibiotics has been advocated for use in these cases, the beads being placed within the bone so that antibiotics can reach the infected bone. Their efficacy has yet to be proved.

For persistently discharging bones, a wide gutter is cut and a skin graft is laid within the gutter (Fig. 4.4).

Salmonella osteomyelitis

Acute osteomyelitis caused by *Salmonella* is found particularly in children who have sickle-cell anaemia. Hence this condition should be looked for if *Salmonella* is present.

Syphilitic osteomyelitis

This disease is uncommon today, as syphilis responds to antibiotics, but in the past two varieties of the infection existed. One, *syphilitic metaphysitis*, affected the metaphysis and produced a picture similar to acute pyogenic osteomyelitis, being found in infants with congenital syphilis. In the second type the infection affects the diaphysis, particularly of the tibia. There is a swelling in the shaft of the bone which may extend the whole length of the bone. Radiologically, the bone has a thickened cortex due to subperiosteal bone formation with an area of bone destruction.

In all cases the Wassermann reaction is positive, which is the feature distinguishing syphilitic osteomyelitis from all other bone infections. Treatment is by administration of a suitable antibiotic.

Tuberculous bone infection

All tuberculous infections in bones and joints are secondary to a tuberculous focus elsewhere, e.g. in the lung, gastrointestinal tract or kidney. Organisms reach the bone or joint through the bloodstream, and the typical feature of this infection is the formation of a "cold" abscess. The abscess tracks its way towards the skin and may then rupture and produce a chronically discharging tuberculous sinus. Joint cartilage is destroyed by proteolytic enzymes produced by the organism, *mycobacterium tuberculosis*.

Mycobacterium tuberculosis is acid-fast on staining with a Ziel Nielsen stain; hence the bacillus is known as the *acid-fast bacillus* (AFB).

Tuberculosis is a generalised disease causing poor general health, weight loss, poor appetite and sometimes a low-grade pyrexia. Effort must be given to seeking a primary focus for the bone infection. The following investigations are required:

1. Blood tests—ESR, full blood count and differential, urea and electrolytes, liver function tests
2. Three consecutive early morning specimens of urine for culture for AFB.
3. Chest X-ray for pulmonary focus
4. Mantoux test
5. Aspiration of joint fluid or needle biopsy of affected bone for AFB culture

Treatment with antibiotics must not be started until an adequate sample has been sent to the laboratory for AFB culture. Absolute bed rest is essential until the disease is under control. An adequate diet should be given, and fortified with vitamins if necessary. The first line treatment with antibiotics is as follows: rifampicin 10 mg/kg per day for children or 600 mg daily for adults, ethambutol 15 mg/kg daily for children and 800 mg daily for adults, and isoniazid (INAH—isonicotinic acid hydrazide) 6 mg/kg in children or 300 mg in adults. This regimen is continued for 3 months, then rifampicin is stopped and ethambutol and isoniazid continued for up to 2 years. Rifampicin has replaced streptomycin because of the latter's ototoxicity to the eighth nerve, causing nerve deafness.

The liver function tests should be repeated periodically when rifampicin is being taken, as hepatitis sometimes occurs. Ethambutol has recently replaced para-amino-salicylic acid (PAS) because PAS caused nausea and vomiting in some cases. Pyridoxine 10 mg daily should be given with isoniazid as this prevents a peripheral neuritis developing with this drug.

Spinal tuberculosis

Bone tuberculosis is seen most frequently in the spine, affecting the vertebral body, although it is also seen in the long bones, the hands and the feet. In the spine the lower thoracic and upper lumbar regions are usually the affected areas. Destruction of the intervertebral disc occurs along with collapse of the anterior aspects of the vertebral bodies on either side; hence two vertebrae are affected in each case. A small erosion is first seen on the X-ray, then gradually more bone is destroyed, along with the intervertebral disc. The spine angulates forwards, producing a marked angulation called a kyphos (Fig. 4.5). The posterior elements of the vertebra are not affected and the spine is therefore stable. A mass of tuberculous tissue develops round the vertebra and is seen on the X-ray as a paraspinal shadow. If no complications occur, the affected vertebrae fuse in the angulated position and the only persisting prob lem is the kyphos, which gives the back an abnormal shape.

Complications of spinal tuberculosis are related to the development of a 'cold' abcess. Should this abscess track back into the spinal canal, conduction along the spinal cord may be affected, and

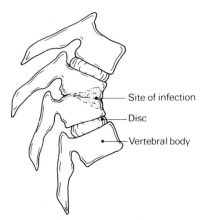

Site of infection

Disc

Vertebral body

Fig. 4.5 Destruction of intervertebral disc and anterior aspect of vertebral body causing angulation of the spine in spinal tuberculosis

a paraplegia may develop (Pott's paraplegia). This is a serious complication, affecting initially muscle power and later sensation. Surgery is necessary to decompress the lesion, and the treatment is described in the section on tuberculosis in Chapter Ten.

Cold abscesses may also track down the psoas muscle and present in the groin below the inguinal ligament, or they may pass down the paravertebral muscles and present in the back. Drainage of the abscess and closure of the incision are necessary to prevent the development of a sinus.

Tuberculous arthritis

Tuberculous arthritis is seen most often in the large joints such as the hip and knee, although any joint may be affected. The presentation is similar to septic arthritis, but there may be a history of exposure to a contact with open tuberculosis. The joint cartilage is rapidly destroyed, and hence early treatment is essential if any of the joint cartilage is to be preserved. Samples of pus are obtained from the joint at open operation and sent for culture. All parts of the investigation noted above should be carried out. After the joint has been decompressed the patient is put on to antituberculous drugs and kept on a regime of strict bed rest. If a hip or knee is affected, traction may be used.

In all cases the tuberculous infection, the patient's overall condition and the ESR are the most helpful indications of the progress of treatment. After about 6 weeks of treatment the patient will become more active and the ESR will be seen to fall. Not until the ESR has fallen to normal limits, however, can the patient be mobilised. Cultures of the samples acquired from the site of infection take at least 6 weeks to incubate, and hence it is only at this late stage that resistant strains can be identified and appropriate changes made in the antibiotic regime.

Septic arthritis

This is a pyogenic infection of a joint and is similar in causation to acute osteomyelitis of the bone. Bloodstream spread is the most common source of the infection, although compound injuries involving the joint can also introduce the infective organism. Spread of infection from a neighbouring osteomyelitis also occurs, particularly where the capsule of the joint encloses some of the metaphysis, as in the hip joint. It is important to identify the causal organism and to decompress a joint under pressure. Open operation is recommended in the obvious case, but where there is doubt needle aspiration as a diagnostic procedure is more appropriate.

A child with septic arthritis appears unwell and refuses to take weight on the affected limb. The involved joint has a restricted range of movement due to pain. There is swelling of the joint—this may not readily be noted in the hip joint, which is located distant from the skin, but in more superficially-placed joints such as the knee swelling is more obvious. As in osteomyelitis the correct antibiotic should be given once the cultures are identified, and the antibiotic should be continued for 3 months.

Delay in treating a septic arthritis will result in serious damage to the articular surface of the joint, and subsequent upon this a fibrous or bony ankylosis may develop.

Five

Bone tumours

Tumours in bone may arise from different types of cell found in bone, and the tumour formed is characteristic of the particular cell type. Thus *osteogenic sarcoma* (*osteosarcoma*) produces new bone which histologically contains a predominance of bone-forming cells. These tumours are known as primary tumours and are either benign or malignant. By far the commonest tumour in bone, however, is the secondary tumour. This arises as a malignant tumour in some other organ in the body and spreads to bone either via the bloodstream or by direct spread. Secondary tumours are malignant, and the common primary sites are breast, lung, prostate, kidney and thyroid (Fig. 5.1).

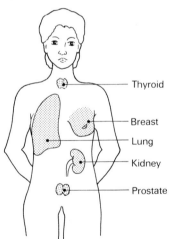

Fig. 5.1 Common sites of primary carcinoma

Presentation of tumours

1. Pain. If a patient who has an established primary tumour in one of the organs listed above, and complains of pain in the back or limb, a secondary tumour in the bone of the affected area should be suspected.

2. Fracture. Similarly, should a patient with a known malignancy fracture a bone, a secondary tumour at the point of the fracture should be suspected.

3. Incidental finding. The routine follow-up of a patient with a malignant tumour that has been treated may reveal an asymptomatic secondary tumour in bone.

4. Swelling. The development of a swelling in a bone or around a joint without a history of trauma may be indicative of primary tumour.

Investigation of a tumour

1. Clinical examination. This is very important to exclude other possible tumours that have not been noticed, and to assess if any spread has occurred.

2. X-rays. Good-quality films of the affected parts are essential, and a chest X-ray should also be taken to exclude pulmonary metatastases.

3. Radio-isotope bone scan. These are valuable in locating other secondary tumours not visible on conventional X-ray films.

4. Computerised axial tomography. Otherwise known as CT scan, this is valuable in assessing local extension of the tumour.

5. Biopsy. This may be performed either by the percutaneous drill biopsy or by open operation removing a piece of the tumour with surrounding tissue for histological examination. If there is a possibility that the lesion may be infective rather than neoplastic, part of the biopsy specimen is sent for bacterial culture.

6. Bone tumour panel. A panel of experts including a surgeon, radiologist, histopathologist, and radiotherapist is available in the centres where a Bone Registry has been established, and the above listed investigations are studied by the panel who suggest the diagnosis and appropriate treatment in patients in whom the diagnosis may be in doubt.

Treatment of bone tumours

Benign tumours

Benign tumours only need treatment if:

1. Their size causes pressure on local structures
2. The tumour involves the juxtarticular part of the epiphysis, and therefore threatens the congruity of the joint surface
3. The tumour involves sufficient bone to render it weak and likely to fracture
4. The diagnosis is in doubt

Treatment involves removal of the tumour if possible, and packing the cavity thus caused by cancellous bone graft.

Malignant primary tumours

The approach to treatment of malignant tumours is very different from that appropriate to the benign type. Open biopsy must be planned with the approach to definitive treatment in mind, particularly the placing of the incision.

The less aggressive tumours may be managed by wide local excision and bridging of the remaining defect with a strut graft (the fibula is a convenient source for the graft). Where a joint is involved a prosthetic replacement can be made with the appropriate joint included. Arthrodesis of the joint is another alternative.

The more aggressive tumours have in the past been treated with amputation and chemotherapy. Trials are in progress using massive prosthetic replacements for these tumours, and the results are awaited with interest. Radiotherapy is only useful in osteosarcomas, as most of the other tumours are resistant to radiotherapy.

Malignant secondary tumours

These are the commonest malignant tumours found in bone. The primary site of the tumour may be the lung, breast, prostate, kidney or thyroid. The patient must be investigated for further lesions in the bone, and the activity of the primary lesion must be assessed. Frequently such tumours are radiosensitive and radiotherapy may be of benefit. Chemotherapy may be used in conjunction with radiotherapy or on its own. Should the tumour involve the shaft of a long bone, and a fracture occur or threaten to occur, an intermedullary nail is inserted. Resection of secondary tumours is rarely

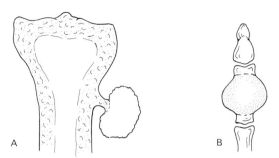

Fig. 5.2 Osteochondromata A) exostosis B) endochrondroma

indicated as their mere presence indicates that the disease is advanced and prognosis poor—although in some cases of carcinoma of the breast where there is a solitary secondary tumour, excision and grafting has been performed.

Common benign tumours

1. Chondrogenic tumours

The *osteochondroma* is a common benign tumour of bone which is characterised by the formation of cartilage. Two types occur, one (*exostosis*) producing an outgrowth from the bone and the other (*enchondroma*) forming within the bone (Fig. 5.2). Diaphysial aclasis is a condition of multiple exostoses and Ollier's disease of multiple enchrondromata.

Much rarer are the benign chondroblastoma and the chondromyxoid fibroma.

2. Osteogenic tumours

These are bone-forming tumours. The *osteoid osteoma* is a small lesion less than 1 cm in diameter and is characterised by being painful but responding to administration of aspirin. The radiographic features consist of a central dense nidus surrounded by a less dense area. Treatment is curettage. Larger tumours are the *osteoblastoma* and *osteoma* (Fig. 5.3).

3. Others

Aneurysmal bone cysts are formed from blood vessel wall and often involve the epiphysis. Distinction from the giant cell tumour

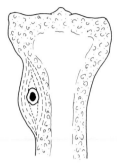

Fig. 5.3 Osteoid osteoma

(osteoclastoma) is difficult, although the latter affects a younger age group. Treatment for both is the same, curettage and grafting, and recurrence is common in both cases. Giant cell tumours occasionally become malignant Fig. 5.4.

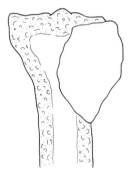

Fig. 5.4 Giant cell tumour

Malignant primary bone tumours

1. Osteogenic tumours

Osteosarcoma is the commonest and most lethal of bone tumours. If affects adolescents and is associated with a low survival rate. It occasionally arises in the elderly in bone affected by Paget's disease. The lesion is identified radiologically by the raised periosteum and Codman's triangle, and sunray spicules (Fig. 5.5). Cade established a treatment regime which consisted of radiotherapy to the tumour; if no lung metastasis occurred after one year amputation of the affected limb was performed, the idea being that if the patient sur-

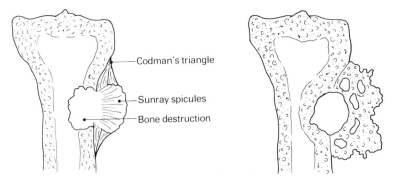

Fig. 5.5 Osteosarcoma

Fig. 5.6 Chondrosarcoma. Blotchy calcification within tumour mass

vived one year without lung secondaries the chance of survival was good enough to merit such a disabling operation. The current trend is to use chemotherapy, and the results are awaited with interest.

2. Chondrogenic tumours

The *chondrosarcoma*, which is comprised of cartilage-forming cells (Fig. 5.6), is less aggressive than the osteosarcoma, and surgical excision is possible in many cases.

3. Others

Fibrosarcoma of bone arises from the fibrous component of the periosteum and bone. It is a bone-destroying (*osteolytic*) tumour and

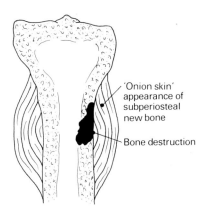

Fig. 5.7 Ewing's tumour

of variable aggressiveness. Surgical ablation combined with radiotherapy and/or chemotherapy is required.

The bone marrow gives rise to two tumours, Ewing's tumour and multiple myeloma. Ewing's tumour affects children and is an aggressive tumour with a poor prognosis. The radiological appearance resembles an 'onion-skin' surrounding the bone (Fig. 5.7). Treatment is by chemotherapy. Multiple myeloma is a tumour of the plasma cells and frequently affects the spine in middle-aged adults. It is characterised by the presence of an abnormal protein (the Bence-Jones protein) in the serum and urine. Chemotherapy again offers the best method of treatment.

Six
Neurological disorders affecting muscle

The nervous system consists of two distinct parts, the central nervous system and the peripheral nerves. Damage to nerves in the central nervous system is irrevocable, as these nerves are unable to regenerate, but in the peripheral nerve regeneration is possible and nerve repair occurs. Details of the physiology and anatomy of the two nervous systems may be found in the companion book in this series, *The Neuromuscular System*.

The central nervous system consists of the brain and the spinal cord. In children the commonest disorders of the upper motor neurone occur in cerebral palsy and spina bifida; in adults a cerebral vascular accident (stroke) is by far the most frequently encountered problem—fractures of the spine and multiple sclerosis are others.

Cerebral palsy

Children with this condition are referred to as being *spastic* because there is increased tone in the muscles and loss of co-ordination. In fact there are five different types of cerebral palsy: 1. Spastic 2. Athetoid 3. Ataxic 4. Rigid 5. Mixed.

Spastic cerebral palsy

In this, the commonest type of cerebral palsy, the affected limb or limbs are held in a characteristic posture—flexed elbow, pronated forearm, flexed wrist for the upper limb, and in the lower limb a flexed knee with plantar flexion at the ankle (Fig. 6.1).

Passive movement of a joint meets with increasing resistance which after a certain point suddenly disappears. Co-ordination is poor in the affected limb, and tendon reflexes may be increased with the presence of clonus.

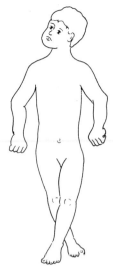

Fig. 6.1 Quadriplegic cerebral palsy. Note adducted hips, scissor gait, equinus feet, clasped hands

In spastic cerebral palsy there is a further subdivision, depending on which limbs are affected:

Monoplegic—affecting one limb only
Diplegic—affecting both lower limbs
Hemiplegic—affecting upper and lower limb on same side
Quadriplegic—affecting all four limbs

Athetoid cerebral palsy

In this condition involuntary movements occur when active movement is commenced, and this is accompanied by variations in the rigidity of joints. No fixed deformity develops. Tendon reflexes are normal.

Ataxic cerebral palsy

This type is a disorder of cerebellar function and is characterised by lack of co-ordination. Muscle tone may be weak and fatigue is common.

Rigid cerebral palsy

This differs from the spastic type because resistance to passive movement occurs immediately on moving a joint and remains throughout the range of movement and after the return of the joint to its original position. The resistance may be *intermittent cogwheel rigidity*, giving the feel of movement against a ratchet, or it may be continuous—*lead-pipe rigity*.

Cerebral palsy is caused by any combination of three factors: premature birth of the fetus, difficulty in labour causing delay or need for assisted delivery, and fetal anoxia.

The assessment of children suffering from cerebral palsy is most important. The paediatrician, neurologist and orthopaedic surgeon should be involved, together with physiotherapists and occupational therapists with an interest in this disorder. The estimation of the intelligence quotient (IQ) must be performed, as many of these children have a low IQ. For a comprehensive study, attendance at a cerebral unit is desirable.

Muscle tone can be reduced by the administration of diazepam or baclofen. If walking is a problem, suitable bracing may be beneficial. Deformity should in the first instance be treated by physiotherapists, but when their treatment fails surgical correction may be indicated.

Hip deformities

Adduction deformity is best treated by an adductor tenotomy and obturator neurectomy (Fig. 6.2). Dividing the adductor muscles allows the fixed adduction to be relieved and division of the obturator nerve (anterior branch only) denervates the adductor muscles and lessens the chance of recurrence of the deformity. Dislocation of the hip may occur as a result of untreated adduction and flexion deformity of the hip. If there is also a rotation deformity, reduction of the hip should be followed by a varus rotation osteotomy, as described in Chapter Eleven.

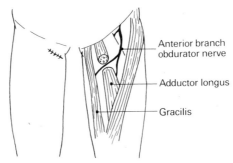

Anterior branch obdurator nerve

Adductor longus

Gracilis

Fig. 6.2 Adductor tenotomy and anterior obdurator neurectomy for adducted hips

Knee deformities

Shortening of the hamstring muscles will cause a flexion deformity of the knee. Where there is minor hamstring shortness the patient is unable to sit up straight with the knees extended, and a proximal hamstring release will overcome this tightness. If a fixed flexion deformity of the knee has developed, release of the hamstrings behind the knee is essential to correct the deformity. Eggers described a distal hamstring release where the hamstring tendons are detached from their insertion in the tibia and reinserted into the distal end of the femur. Many variations on this theme have been described (Fig. 6.3).

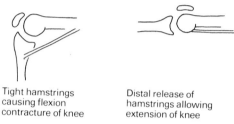

Tight hamstrings
causing flexion
contracture of knee

Distal release of
hamstrings allowing
extension of knee

Fig. 6.3 Eggers distal hamstring release

Ankle deformities

Equinus is the commonest deformity, and if noticed early should be controlled by a physiotherapist. Should a fixed deformity develop, elongation of the Achilles tendon, preferably by the slide technique, should correct it. The tendon is partially divided medially proximally, and distally it is partially divided anteriorly. The foot is plantar flexed and the tendon fibres unwind allowing the tendon to

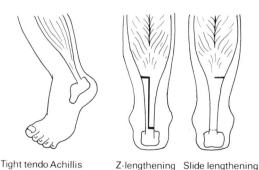

Tight tendo Achillis   Z-lengthening   Slide lengthening

Fig. 6.4 Correction of equinus foot in cerebral palsy by surgical release of the tendo Achillis

elongate. No sutures are required in the tendon; the skin is closed and a plaster applied for 6 weeks, after which the child is readmitted to hospital for intensive mobilisation. Alternatively, the tendon can be formally lengthened using the Z-technique (Fig. 6.4).

Spina bifida

This condition is considered at length in Chapter Ten. Failure of development of the spinal column at any level may result in failure of the nerve supply. The area normally innervated by the affected nerve or nerves therefore lacks both sensation and motor power. As spina bifida is a congenital abnormality, the affected part fails to grow at the normal rate, and urinary and bowel control are frequently affected.

Cerebral vascular accidents

These are common in the elderly and may consist of a cerebral thrombosis or haemorrhage. In the younger adult a subarachnoid haemorrhage may produce a similar clinical picture. Treatment from the orthopaedic point of view is limited to the treatment of residual deformity or paralysis long after the acute stage of the disease has passed. External splintage is usually all that is required. Surgery is only rarely undertaken and may be linked with anxiety on the part of both patient and surgeon that a further cerebrovascular accident may occur.

Fractures of the spine

Fracture-dislocation of the spine may cause irreversible damage to the spine should the spinal cord be compressed or the blood supply to the spine be interrupted (Fig. 6.5). If the fracture-dislocation occurs high in the cervical spine and the function of the cord is lost distally from that point, the patient will die of a respiratory arrest at the time of the injury. Lesions in the mid-cervical spine cause a quadriplegia, which is a paralysis of all four limbs associated with sensory loss. Respiration in quadriplegia is maintained by the phrenic nerve (C3, 4, 5,) and is hence diaphragmatic. Lower cervical lesions cause a partial paralysis of the upper limbs and a complete paralysis of the lower limbs.

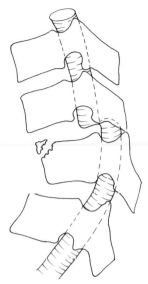

Fig. 6.5 Fracture-dislocation of spine, showing mechanism of damage to spinal cord

Thoracic fractures produce a paraplegia—paralysis of the lower limbs and the lower the fracture the less extensive the nerve damage. Because the upper motor neurone is damaged, there is no hope of regeneration of the damaged nerves. The bladder and anal sphincter are innervated by nerves from the pelvic plexus. These are autonomic nerves from both the sympathetic and parasympathetic nervous system. The sympathetic component comes from T 12 to L 2 and the parasympathetic from S 2 to S 4 in the nervi erigentes. The sympathetic nerves operate the sphincters of the bladder and anus whereas the parasympathetics operate the emptying muscles, the detrusor muscle of the bladder and the muscles of the descending and sigmoid colon.

Following injury to the spinal cord there is a period of time that may last only 48 hours or up to 6 weeks which is called spinal shock. This is the result of the cord being stretched at the time of the injury. The limbs are flaccid and the bladder and rectum paralysed. As soon as this stage is passed, return of reflex activity occurs, causing spastic paralysis to develop. The slightest stimulation to the skin in the affected region may cause a massive contraction of the muscles by reflex arcs.

The bladder will develop reflex emptying if the spinal cord is damaged above the segments of the cord where the bladder reflex passes, i.e. above S 2, which is found in the lumbar enlargement of the cord lying in the adult between the vertebral bodies of T. 10 and L. 1. As urine distends the bladder, the stretch receptors become active and cause reflex emptying of the bladder.

Should this reflex be broken by the spinal injury, the bladder remains flaccid, and although a nerve plexus within the wall of the bladder can stimulate it to contract, this contraction is localised and is not sufficient to empty the bladder. This can only be achieved by external compression or the use of an indwelling catheter. An ileal bladder may be constructed in these cases.

The reflex bladder is known as an *automatic bladder*, the non-reflex type the *autonomous bladder*, and the bladder during the time of spinal shock the *neurogenic bladder*.

Nursing care is by far the most important facet in the management of spinal injuries. Patients often die from infection having overcome the immediate effects of the spinal injury. Infection may take the form of pneumonia, infected pressure sores or urinary tract infection.

Pneumonia in these patients is of the hypostatic type caused by inadequate turning and chest physiotherapy. Pressure sores occur rapidly unless the patient is nursed correctly, because the skin is anaesthetic, and ischaemic necrosis develops if the pressure areas are not relieved by turning the patient every 2 hours. Treating the pressure points by washing gently with soap and water, incorporating gentle massage and applying oil if the skin is dry, is essential. Urinary tract infections arise from bacteria entering the bladder along the side of a catheter, and strict aseptic precautions are required when catheterising these patients. Where possible, intermittent self catheterisation is taught; if the bladder cannot be trained, then an indwelling catheter is required. In either case, frequent specimens of urine should be sent for culture.

A conventional bed is adequate for nursing patients with spinal injuries, providing that a soft foam or Sorbo mattress is available (Fig. 6.6). The patient is nursed on pillows placed beneath the loin

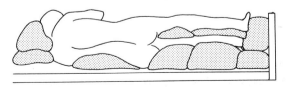

Fig. 6.6 Method of nursing paraplegic patient on pillows

and legs and the heels are protected with sheepskin or other suitable pads. The patient must be turned regularly every 2 hours, and no nursing procedure must be allowed to disrupt this routine. Turning should be controlled so that no rotational strain is placed across the fracture. A motorised tilting bed has been designed at Stoke Mandeville Hospital. It can tilt the patient on to either side with very little effort and is available in some centres.

The surgical management of spinal fractures is determined by the level of the fracture and whether it is stable. Unstable cervical fractures are managed on traction. Crutchfield tongs or other caliper are applied to the skull and a weight is suspended over a pulley at the head of the bed. It is important that when turning these patients the cervical spine is moved as the thoracolumbar spine is turned. As soon as any residual dislocation has reduced a Minerva jacket or a halo-body vest is applied. Gross instability may require spinal fusion. If the fracture is stable and displacement absent or minimal a cervical collar alone may be sufficient.

The cervical spine is much more mobile than the thoracolumbar spine, and hence fracture-dislocations in the latter region require greater force and the local damage is proportionately greater. Unstable fractures require stabilisation either to prevent a partial lesion becoming completer or to aid the nursing care of the patient. Surgical stabilisation in this region is best performed by posterior fusion, either using plates along the spinous processes or introducing the Harrington rod as used in the correction of scoliosis. Bone graft is placed over the laminae.

After the initial treatment has been established, attention should be directed to the mobilisation of the patient and his rehabilitation. Practical problems such as the establishment of micturition need to be resolved along the lines already suggested. Bowel actions can usually be initiated by abdominal straining and the use of aperients and bulk purgatives. Manual removal of faeces should only be required in the early phase of the treatment. An ileal bladder may need to be constructed if the patient has an autonomous bladder.

The physiotherapist must develop what muscle power remains. In the quadriplegic there is unlikely to be any useful muscle power in the upper limbs, and he may need considerable support for the rest of his life, but the paraplegic should have normal power in the upper limbs and efforts to get him mobile, on crutches if possible, are made. Resettlement in employment within the physical capabilities of the patient is then undertaken.

Poliomyelitis

Acute anterior poliomyelitis is caused by a virus which gains access to the body through the nasopharynx or alimentary tract. This condition is now rare due to a very effective immunisation campaign. The acute phase begins with a generalised illness, after which paralysis occurs in certain muscle groups. The virus lodges in the anterior horn cell of the spinal cord and if the cell is damaged paralysis of the supplied muscle develops (Fig. 6.7). Sensation, however, is not affected. In the acute phase a lumbar puncture and analysis of the cerebrospinal fluid are necessary to confirm the diagnosis.

In the acute phase the patient is nursed in bed and the affected limbs are gently put through a passive range of movements. Not until the acute phase is passed is the patient mobilised, because premature mobilisation is said to be associated with a worse prognosis. The orthopaedic surgeon becomes involved when deformity arises, but with good physiotherapy contractures should not occur. As this disease affects children, however, bone growth will be affected in severe cases and the child may present many years after the infection with a short leg. Walking is the priority in the management of these patients. A severely affected leg may have no active muscle power, yet the patient may be able to walk. On close inspection the foot may be found to be in fixed equinus and the leg shorter than the unaffected side. Walking is then achieved by extending the knee into hyperextension (the so-called *back kneeing*) by extension of the hip, either using gluteus maximus or by using the upper limb to force the femur backwards, so that the knee locks in extension. The equinus, providing that it is no more than 20°, helps the knee to hyperextend. A patient with this combination of deformities should be able to walk unaided, and no surgery is indicated.

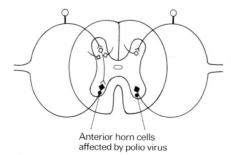

Anterior horn cells
affected by polio virus

Fig. 6.7 Diagrammatic illustration of the action of polio virus on the spinal cord

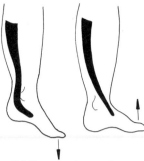

Fig. 6.8 Transfer of the tibialis posterior tendon to achieve dorsi-flexion of the foot

Should a flexion deformity develop at the knee, it needs to be corrected so that the knee can be extended. The most effective way of correcting this is by supracondylar osteotomy of the femur. Marked equinus is best managed with a Lambrinudi pan talar arthrodesis. A wedge is removed from the talus on its underside so that the equinus is corrected. Other forms of arthrodesis are also used.

Tendons that remain active can be re-routed to perform the function of paralysed muscles. The commonest tendon transfer is the tibialis posterior transfer to a paralysed tibialis anterior (Fig. 6.8). The tibialis posterior tendon is passed through the intermuscular septum of the lower limb and sutured to the dorsum of the foot to produce dorsi-flexion. All transferred tendons tend to lose some power; a muscle power 5 becomes power 4. It is important to record accurately a muscle chart of the affected limb before any treatment is undertaken, and a careful study of limb function is essential.

There are many splints that have been used in polio patients, and some of the latest cosmetic calipers in particular are a great improvement on the traditional designs. The cosmetic caliper is basically a gutter splint that is held against the back of the limb and includes the foot. It is made of a robust material and hence it can be fairly thin and unobtrusive. The splint passes around the heel and provides a very adequate toe raising effect without any of the traditional springs and straps. Worn under tights it is hardly noticeable.

The spine may develop a paralytic scoliosis if it is affected, and correction and fusion may be required as described in Chapter Ten.

The management of polio after the acute phase has passed may be summarised as follows:

1. Thorough assessment
2. Correction of fixed flexion deformity
3. Splintage where necessary
4. Tendon transfer where possible
5. Enabling patient to walk, or if this is not possible provision of aids to give maximum mobility

Brachial plexus lesions

Traction injury of the cervical nerves in the neck may produce a variety of lesions. The nerve roots may be avulsed from the spinal cord (preganglionic lesion) or they may rupture at any point in the brachial plexus (postganglionic lesion). The brachial plexus is made up of the cervical nerves C5, C6, C7 and C8 and the first thoracic, T1. These roots group into trunks, the upper containing C5 and C6, the middle C7 and the lower C8 and T1. These trunks then divide into anterior and posterior divisions. The anterior division of the upper and middle trunks form the lateral cord, the anterior division of the lower trunk continues as the medial cord and the posterior cord is made up of all the posterior divisions. From the lateral cord arises the median nerve, from the medial cord the ulnar nerve and from the posterior the radial nerve. For the branches of the brachial plexus see Fig. 6.9.

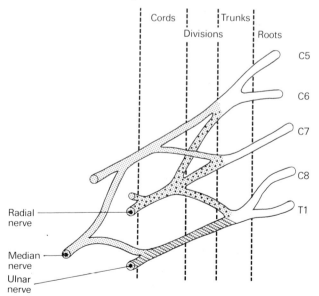

Fig. 6.9 Divisions of the brachial plexus

Injuries to these nerves occur when the head is pressed to one side and the shoulder depressed as when a motocyclist is thrown from his machine and his head hits the ground and is forced to one side, allowing the shoulder to hit the ground in its turn and be depressed. The nerves are forcibly stretched and damage occurs. If the nerves are avulsed from the spinal cord there is no hope of recovery, as the nerves cannot regenerate within the spinal cord. Lesions distal to the ganglion on the dorsal root may involve a total rupture (*neurotmesis*), or the nerve sheath may remain intact while the axon within it is divided (*axonotmesis*), or the nerve may be stretched without organic rupture of its components although transmission of nerve impulses is temporarily inhibited (*neuropraxia*) (Fig.6.10). Nerve regeneration may occur across a neurotemesis provided that the divided nerve-ends are closely approximated, but recovery will depend on how well new axons develop and the state of the neural tubes of the distal nerve stump. In axonotemis nerve regeneration should occur along the correct nerve sheath producing good recovery, provided that there is little intraneural fibrosis. Neuropraxias recover rapidly usually with only minimal loss of nerve conduction if any.

A brachial plexus lesion is suspected in a patient who has sustained major trauma to the upper limbs and neck. The limb will be numb (paraesthetic) and active movement in muscles innervated by the injured nerves will be paralysed. Severe injuries may be associated with a Horner's syndrome, which implies damage to the cervical sympathetic fibres and avulsion of nerve roots from the cord.

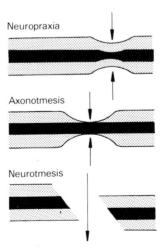

Fig. 6.10 Different kinds of nerve injury

In Horner's syndrome the pupil on the affected side is smaller than the opposite pupil and will not dilate. The patient may have other injuries, such as fractures.

Assessment includes a good muscle chart and X-rays of the cervical spine. In the early stages exploration of the injured plexus may be helpful, as any repair that might be possible has a better prognosis at this stage. Prior to surgery myelography may be useful in showing avulsed roots as meningeal pouches around the myodil. Electrical conduction in the limb and from the limb to the cerebral cortex will help in differentiating between ruptured nerves and lesions in continuity.

Nerves regenerate at a rate of one millimetre a day and hence recovery takes many months. Meanwhile it is important to keep joints mobile and to provide suitable splintage so that the patient can use the affected limb. If the limb is totally paralysed (flail arm) a flail arm splint is supplied. This will hold the elbow flexed and there are a variety of gadgets that can be attached to the wrist portion, such as a hook, so that the splint can complement the function of the normal limb. Splints are arranged so that movements of the opposite shoulder will initiate opening and closing of attachments fixed to the splint. Rehabilitation is very important, and employers need encouragement to employ these patients.

Erb palsy

This is an injury to the upper trunk of the brachial plexus that occurs during birth, caused by the shoulder being depressed. If it fails to recover, the shoulder becomes fixed in internal rotation, forearm in pronation, held behind the back with the palm facing upwards, (the waiter's position).

Klumpke palsy

Like the Erb palsy this is a birth injury. The arm is forcibly elevated during birth causing injury to the lower trunk of the plexus. Paralysis is found in the forearm and hand. Many of these birth injuries recover spontaneously; those that do not develop secondary contractures of the soft tissues.

Peripheral nerve lesions

As outlined in the previous section nerve injuries are classified as:

1. Neuropraxia
2. Axonotmesis
3. Neurotmesis

Electrical nerve conduction and electromyographic studies will help differentiate between axonotmesis and neuropraxia. Neuropraxias may recover within hours of the injury. Repair of divided nerves should be performed within 3 months of the injury for optimum results. There was formerly a practice of delayed suture of nerves, waiting for local damage to the nerve to be revealed by the presence of fibrosis and then re-exploring the nerves at 6 weeks, but the present practice of many is to perform early primary repair of the divided nerve, as the longer the time interval between injury and repair the greater the chance for fibrous tissue to grow down the neural tubes of the distal stump, preventing any future nerve regeneration. Nerve surgery is increasingly being performed with the aid of magnification, particularly using the operating microscope. This allows very fine suture material to be used, and approximation of the nerve fascicles is possible. If the outer covering of the nerve is used for the suture, the suture is *epineural*, if fascicles are sutured together the suture is *perineural*. Large gaps in the nerve can be bridged by nerve grafts. These are either isolated, taking a nerve such as the sural, or vascularised, where the blood supply to the graft is connected to blood vessels adjacent to the nerve defect. Pedicle grafts may be used when two adjacent nerves are divided. In the forearm the ulnar nerve can be used as a pedicle graft. Initially, the proximal cut ends of both nerves are sutured to each other, and 6 weeks later the ulnar nerve is divided high in the forearm, the cut end being brought distally to be sutured to the distal stump of the median nerve, retaining the blood supply to the graft. This allows restoration in the median nerve after regeneration of the nerve fibres, but no recovery can occur in the ulnar nerve.

Axillary nerve paralysis

The axillary nerve was formerly termed the circumflex nerve. It winds around the neck of the humerus and is damaged in dislocation of the shoulder. The deltoid is paralysed and there is a loss of sensation over the insertion of that muscle. Shoulder movements must be maintained during recovery of the nerve, which usually takes from 2 to 6 months.

Median nerve paralysis

This nerve can be damaged at any point in its course. If the damage occurs in the arm or elbow, paralysis of the long flexors of the wrist and fingers occurs with sensory loss over the lateral three and one half fingers, whereas division of the nerve in the lower forearm and wrist causes loss of sensation but only paralysis of the abductor pollicis brevis.

Ulnar nerve paralysis

Lesions of this nerve in the arm or in the ulnar groove behind the elbow produce loss of sensation over the medial one and one half fingers with paralysis of the wrist flexor on the ulnar side and the long flexors to the ring and little fingers. The small muscles of the hand are paralysed apart from the thumb short abductor. Lesions at the wrist are similar with the exception that the long flexors and wrist flexor are spared. Unfortunately, penetrating injuries at the wrist damage not only nerves but also the adjacent tendons and arteries.

Radial nerve paralysis

The radial nerve winds around the shaft of the humerus between the lateral and medial heads of the triceps muscle. The nerve is readily damaged in fractures of the mid shaft of the humerus. Paralysis of the wrist and finger extensors results, with sensory loss over the dorsum of the thumb, index and middle finger. At the wrist the superfical radial nerve lies over the lateral side of the forearm, and if damaged produces an area of sensory loss in this distribution.

Hand nerve lesions

The median nerve passes through the carpal tunnel and may become compressed, giving rise to the carpal tunnel syndrome. The patient wakes at night with pain in the hand with altered sensation in the lateral three and one half fingers. Elevating the hand relieves the symptoms. The condition is easily rectified by decompressing the carpal tunnel, dividing the roof of this tunnel in the palm. The procedure is frequently performed on an outpatient basis.

The ulnar nerve branches in the hand into the deep branch, which is motor to the small muscles of the hand, and sensory branches. The deep branch may be divided as an isolated injury by penetrating injuries. This would lead to a paralysis of the small muscles and subsequent wasting.

The digital nerves are easily divided in association with lacerations to the lateral aspects of the fingers. If the digital nerve to the lateral aspect of the index finger is damaged, considerable disability occurs, and repair is desirable. The use of the operating microscope is a distinct advantage.

Reconstructive surgery

Nerve repairs that have failed to provide sufficient re-innervation of muscles, or nerve lesions that have remained untreated for two years require tendon transfer to regain function. The basic scheme of tendon transfer is as follows:

High median nerve lesion. The extensor carpi radialis longus tendon is rerouted into the flexor pollicis longus and the flexor digitorum profundus of the ring finger is rerouted into the profundus tendon of the index finger.

Ulnar nerve lesion. The extensor pollicis brevis is rerouted to the first dorsal interosseous and a Zancolli performed on the flexor digitorum sublimis to correct the clawing of the fingers, part of the tendon being brought back and over the tendon sheath to act as a lasso.

Radial nerve lesion. The flexor carpi ulnaris tendon is put into the extensor digitorum comminus and the extensor pollicis longus, the pronator teres is transfered into the extensor carpi radialis brevis and the palmaris longus into the abductor pollicis longus.

Lower limb nerve lesions

Sciatic nerve paralysis

Damage to this nerve arises as a complication of fractures of the pelvis, traumatic dislocation of the hip and operations around the hip joint and is also associated with fractures of the femur. If the lesion is complete there is paralysis of all muscles below the knee, with sensory loss. If the nerve is believed to be divided it is explored and sutured as necessary. Insensitive skin must be protected and the joints of the foot and ankle kept mobile to prevent trophic ulcers and fixed deformity occurring. A caliper with toe-raising facility should be worn while awaiting recovery of the nerve.

Peroneal nerve paralysis (lateral popliteal nerve)

This nerve arises from the sciatic nerve and winds around the neck of the fibula. In this position it is close to the skin and vulnerable. Fractures of the fibula or compression from a tightly fitting plaster cast can cause damage to the nerve at this point. A foot drop develops, associated with loss of sensation over the lateral aspect of the leg and dorsum of the foot. The drop foot requires a toe-raising spring and caliper, or a gutter cosmetic toe-raising splint which is worn under a sock inside the shoe.

Postoperative care

All nerve repairs are protected where possible in a plaster cast for 6 weeks. Tendon transfer in the upper limb are immobilised in plaster for 3 weeks, and patients are then readmitted for intensive physiotherapy and re-education of tendon function. Sensory re-education plays an important part in the rehabilitation of the patient and is performed when sensation is returning to the affected part. Painful neuromata respond in many cases to transcutaneous electrical stimulation.

Seven

Common fractures

Fractures are classified either as *transverse, oblique* or *spiral*, and the bone is divided into a *proximal* and a *distal* fragment or the fracture may be described as *comminuted* when the bone is fractured into three or more pieces. If the skin is intact the fracture is *closed* and there is no danger of infection of the fracture through the skin, but if the skin is lacerated over the fracture, the fracture is exposed and termed *compound*. In children the bones are soft, and the bone tends to buckle, forming a *greenstick fracture*. It is essential to determine the details of how the fracture was sustained to understand the dynamics of injury. Direct blows tend to cause transverse fractures, twisting injuries cause spiral fractures and major injuries lead to compound fractures. (See Fig. 7.1.)

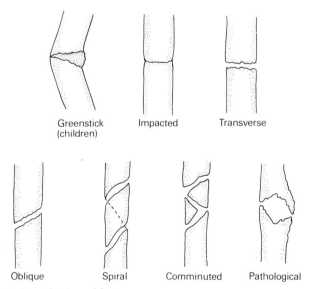

Greenstick (children)   Impacted   Transverse

Oblique   Spiral   Comminuted   Pathological

Fig. 7.1 Classification of fractures

Initial management

The limb should be assessed for signs of external damage and the pulses felt for to establish the state of the circulation. If the circulation is impaired and the limb grossly angulated at the fracture, gentle correction of the deformity may restore the circulation. The limb should be splinted before the patient is moved—the ambulance service has a wide variety of splints, the most commonly used being the inflatable type. On arrival at the hospital the clothes are removed from the injured limb, care being taken not to disturb the fracture. Clothes are best cut rather than pulled. The circulation to the limb is then reassessed, and any skin lacerations are covered with a light gauze dressing. The patient should not be given anything by mouth in case there is a need for a general anaesthetic. The patient's property should be cared for in the standard way, and consideration should be given to the relatives, who should wait in a suitable place while preliminary management is taking place.

Examination of patient

The doctor will need to examine the whole of the patient, and he will depend on you to maintain as much privacy as is possible in the circumstances. The patient will be X-rayed and blood samples will be taken. Pressure area care is important at this stage, particularly if there is likely to be a wait between the special investigations and the warding of the patient. Let the doctor know that relatives are waiting so that he may speak to them. Ventfoam traction may be required for lower limb fractures, and details of its application are to be found in Chapter Fourteen, as are the details for plaster application. The doctor will require the neurological examination tray to complete his examination. Continually reassure the patient that the doctor's examination and the immediate special investigations are important, and that treatment will follow after a full assessment. Baseline observations should be performed by the nurse during this investigative phase: these include TPR and BP together with observation of circulation in the affected limb, skin colour, temperature and pulses. Where indicated, a head injury chart should be used.

Treatment of fractures

The basic principle for the immobilisation of fractures has always

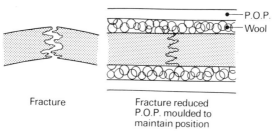

Fig. 7.2 Treatment of fractures with a plaster of Paris cast

been to immobilise the limb from the joint above the fracture to the joint below the fracture. Thus a forearm fracture is splinted from the upper arm to the hand, the elbow and wrist being immobilised. Plaster of Paris in bandage form has been used for the last two centuries as the splint, and only recently have newer synthetic materials been produced. The plaster is applied and moulded while still wet and pliable, using the three point fixation principle. Pressure is applied at the fracture site to correct angular deformity, and pressure is applied on the opposite side of the plaster cast as far distant from the fracture as possible (Fig. 7.2). The term 'cast' is now used instead of 'plaster' because of the advent of newer materials: the 'plaster' is therefore called a plaster cast, whereas a cast made of the synthetic material Hexelite is a Hexelite cast. After the application and trimming of the cast, it is laid on pillows until dry, which for plaster of Paris may take up to 48 hours, whereas synthetic casts harden in 20 minutes. Weight-bearing is only allowed if the fracture permits and the cast is dry. Patients can be classified as *non-weight bearing* when they need to walk with crutches, *partial weight-bearing* when weight-bearing is allowed provided crutches are used when the affected limb touches the ground, or *full weight-bearing* when no external aid is necessary. Details of nursing care of plaster casts are to be found in Chapter Fourteen.

Fractures below the elbow or below the knee are usually immobilised in a cast. The fractures above the elbow usually are usually best managed in a collar and cuff or a sling. Fractures of the femur require traction for at least six weeks, after which a cast-brace may be applied. This is a specialised technique in casting, involving the application of a skin-tight cast and using hinges at the knee.

Specific fracture treatment

1. Shoulder girdle and humerus

A collar and cuff is usually sufficient to control these fractures. A sling applied over the collar and cuff may be helpful in the first few days by taking some of the weight of the forearm. Observe for impaired circulation in the forearm and hand, and note any swelling. Encourage the patient to more the fingers frequently. Check the sensation in the hand together with the radial pulse. Details of the different fractures are in Chapter Eight.

2. Forearm and wrist

Details of these fractures are to be found in Chapter Nine. Plaster casts are applied, above elbow for fractures of the forearm and below elbow for fractures of the wrist. Fractures of the wrist are often associated with swelling of the hand, and elevation of the plaster cast in a high sling is important in the first 48 hours. Swelling in the hand impedes movement of the fingers, and compression of the medial nerve at the wrist also occasionally occurs as the result of swelling, hence the importance of high elevation. Persistent swelling of the fingers with lack of use predisposes to Sudeck's atrophy, which delays healing of the fracture and causes considerable disability (see Chapter Nine).

3. Fingers and hand

Fractures of the fingers involving the proximal and middle phalanges are best managed with bridge strapping, the fractured finger being

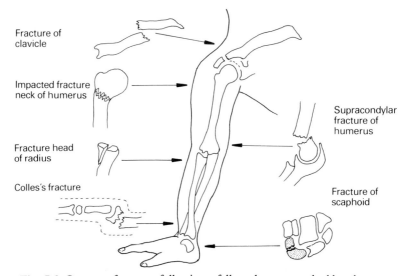

Fig. 7.3 Common fractures following a fall on the outstretched hand

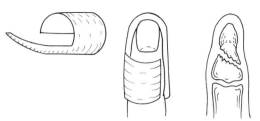

Fig. 7.4 Fracture of the terminal phalanx and the Oakley mallet splint

strapped to an adjacent unfractured finger. This allows movement at the joints, which usually corrects any rotational deformity. Fractures of the distal phalanx are best treated with a mallet splint, the most satisfactory being the Oakley splint (Fig. 7.4). Fractures of the metacarpals occur as a spiral fracture of the shaft or a fracture at the neck (Fig. 7.5). Rotational deformity needs to be corrected or the finger will not flex in the same plane as the other fingers. A slab of plaster moulded around the palm maintains the position.

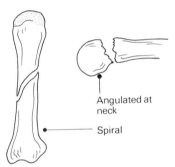

Angulated at neck

Spiral

Fig. 7.5 Fractures of the metacarpal

4. Spine

See Chapter Ten.

5. Pelvis (fig vii. 6 & 7)

Minor fractures, such as isolated pubic ramus fractures, need only symptomatic treatment. Major fractures either cause disruption to the pelvic rim with damage to the sacroiliac joints, often involving damage to soft tissues within the pelvis such as the urethra, or occur around the acetabulum, where the weight-bearing part of the pelvis from the sacrum to the femur fractures. Two thick columns of bone pass between these bones, one anterior and one posterior.

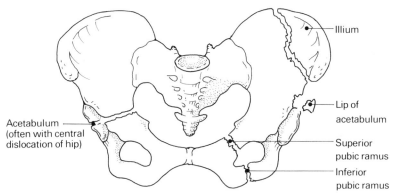

Fig. 7.6 Isolated pelvic fractures

Dislocation of the hip, either centrally into the pelvis or posteriorly, may also occur (Figs 7.6 and 7.7).

The first type of fracture, with the pelvic rim opened out, is best treated with the pelvis suspended in a sling. Obviously, any injury to the pelvic contents also requires treatment. Treatment of fractures of the anterior and posterior columns usually require internal fixation, usually with screws, and avulsed fragments of the acetabulum can be accurately reduced. Dislocation of the hip posteriorly reduces readily with manipulation, but central dislocations with fracture of the acetabulum require skeletal traction to reduce the fracture, usually for 6 weeks followed by a further 6 weeks of non-weight-bearing on crutches.

6. Upper end of femur

These fractures are either through the neck of the femur or around

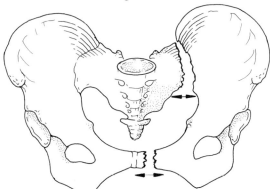

Fig. 7.7 Fractures with disruption of the pelvic rim

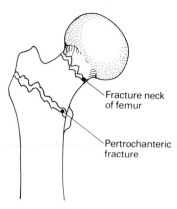

Fracture neck
of femur

Pertrochanteric
fracture

Fig. 7.8 Fractures of the upper end of the femur

the trochanter (the *pertrochanteric* fractures) (Fig. 7.8). Slightly displaced fractures of the neck of the femur are internally fixed with a
nail or nail and plate, whereas severely displaced fractures are
treated with replacement using an Austin Moore or a Thompson
prosthesis because the head of the femur in such cases is likely to be
devoid of a blood supply (see Chapter Eleven). Fractures around
the trochanters are treated with a pin and plate or one of the newer
deriviatives of this technique (sliding screw and plate).

7. Femoral shaft

Shaft fractures of the femur have been treated for centuries with
traction. This method relies on the body forming callus around the
fracture in sufficient quantities to provide a stable bond between
the broken ends of the bone. This process in adults takes around 12
weeks, a little less for spiral fractures and a little more for transverse fractures. In children the time required is half that of adults.
Several methods of applying traction have been devised; the commonest are Hamilton-Russell traction, sliding traction using a Thomas splint, and fixed traction. In children, gallows traction is ideal
for those under one year old and a straight pull with the foot of the
bed elevated is suitable for those over one year old (Fig. 7.9).

Internal fixation of femoral shaft fractures, if performed on a
suitable fracture, will enable a patient to become mobile after about
2 weeks and hence to be allowed home, preventing the long stay in
hospital that is associated with treatment on traction. Transverse
fractures are treated with intramedullary nails, and oblique fractures with a plate. There are disadvantages to internal fixation
which must not be forgotten (p. 5).

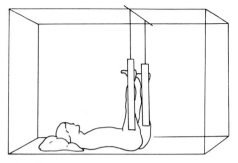

Fig. 7.9 Gallows traction

Recently, cast bracing has become popular. This involves the application of a cast that is so shaped that it transmit the body weight from the limb above the fracture to the cast, bypassing the fracture to a large extent. In femoral cast bracing a hinge is applied at the knee to allow flexion but prevent rotation. These casts may be applied as soon as the fracture becomes stable, i.e. at about 6 weeks for femoral shaft fractures.

8. Fractures around the knee

Fractures of the lower femur involving the knee joint will require internal fixation with a blade plate unless the fracture is undisplaced and fairly stable (Fig. 7.10). Fractures of the upper end of the tibia require reduction if they are displaced and involve the knee joint. The reduction can be achieved either by mobilising the knee on a Braun frame or by electing internal fixation as primary treatment. Such fractures in adults usually unite in 6 weeks. Fractures of the patella, if undisplaced, need treatment in a plaster cylinder for 6 weeks, but if displaced they necessitate reduction of the fragments and repair of the patellar retinaculum using tension band wiring (Fig. 7.11). Badly comminuted fractures are best treated with patellectomy. Ligamentous injuries associated with these fractures should be managed as described in Chapter Twelve.

9. Tibia

Tibial shaft fractures usually unite between 6 and 8 weeks. The lower the fracture the slower the union, and this is particularly so in the distal third of the tibia where non-union is not uncommon. Usually, these fractures can be adequately treated with closed reduction and an above knee plaster, perhaps applying a cast brace at

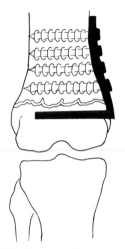

Fig. 7.10 Supracondylar fracture of the femur fixed with blade plate

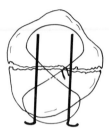

Fig. 7.11 Fracture of the patella fixed with tension band wiring

four weeks. Intramedullary nailing or plate fixation may be indicated if the fracture is difficult to reduce. All fractures of the tibia must be admitted to hospital for elevation for at least 48 hours as they tend to cause swelling, and Volkmann's ischaemic contracture may develop if the swelling is unchecked. If the fracture is well reduced and stable, partial weight-bearing can be allowed, but if the fracture is unstable the patient is mobilised non-weight-bearing.

10. Ankle

Fractures of the ankle are often referred to as *Pott's fracture*. This can be very confusing as there are several types of fracture, and the type of the fracture is directly related to the mechanism of injury.

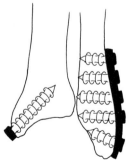

Fig. 7.12 Fracture of the ankle fixed with plate and compression screw

Closed reduction of ankle fractures is satisfactory where only one malleolus is fractured, but bimalleolar fractures are usually unstable and require fixation with a screw or small plate. Disruption of the inferior tibio-fibular joint requires reduction and fixation, as do ligament ruptures (Fig. 7.12). Minor fractures of the ankle, after the application of a below-knee plaster, can be allowed home non-weight-bearing until the plaster has dried, and partial weight-bearing thereafter. The fracture is usually united at 6 weeks when the plaster is removed and the fracture X-rayed. Mobilisation of the joint may require treatment in the physiotherapy department for a few weeks. Severe fractures must be admitted to hospital for elevation and reduction.

11. Foot

Metatarsal fractures (*march fractures*) are common, and only require a below-knee cast, if painful, for 3 to 6 weeks. Multiple fractures due to violent injury are associated with swelling and haemorrhage. These require admission to hospital and elevation until the swelling has resolved. A plaster cast can then be applied.

12. Jaw and face (*mandible and maxilla*)

These fractures are included because they often occur with multiple injuries and demand skilled nursing care. Fractures of the mandible are immobilised with interdental wiring when teeth are present and where there are no teeth (edentulous), circumferential wiring or a Gunning splint is used. External fixation with a splint is also possible. Sepsis is always a potential complication of such fractures, and preventative measures include careful oral hygiene and the administration of antibiotics. Only liquids can be given, so a balanced liquidised diet should be arranged. Fractures of the maxilla are classified

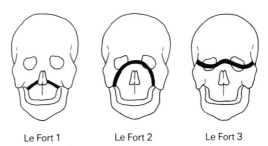

Le Fort 1   Le Fort 2   Le Fort 3

Fig. 7.13 Classification of maxillary fractures

into three groups following the system of Le Fort. Le Fort I is a fracture that separates the maxilla from the rest of the facial bones; Le Fort II extends to the inner side of both orbits; and Le Fort III is a complete separation of the facial bones from the rest of the skull (Fig. 7.13). The fractures are readily recognised on X-ray. Leakage of cerebrospinal fluid through the nose *rhinorrhoea* is common and must be treated with antibiotics to prevent infection. Treatment of Le Fort fractures consists of immobilising the maxilla by fixing it to the skull, and this is usually done with pins and a frame. Fractures of the malar-zygomatic region, involving the zygomatic arch and the inferior orbital plate, are often depressed and require elevation and fixation.

Classification of fractures

1. Closed
2. Compound
3. Complicated

Fractures may be *simple*, the bone being broken into two parts, the fracture line being *transverse*, *oblique* or *spiral*, or they may be *comminuted* where three or more parts have been produced. If the skin is broken over the fracture the fracture is *compound*. If the skin was broken by the bone being forced through the skin the puncture wound in the skin may be small, whereas if the skin was lacerated the wound will be larger. In all compound injuries the wound must be cleaned surgically and debris removed in aseptic conditions. *Complicated fractures* are fractures where there has been associated injury to a nerve or major blood vessel at the site of the injury.

Classification of treatment

1. Closed manipulation and application of external cast (plaster)
2. Open reduction with internal fixation (plates, screws and nails)
3. Closed intramedullary nailing (under X-ray control without disturbing the fracture site)

Fracture healing

Details of this process are given in Chapter One. If the process progresses until the fracture is sound, *union* is said to have occurred. If the healing process is slow *delayed union* is said to have occurred and additional forms of fixation may be required; bone grafting may even be considered. *Non-union* occurs when dense fibrous tissue bridges the fracture and there is no evidence of new bone formation. In non-union, bone grafting is necessary to establish union. Recently, an electrical current passed across the fracture site has been tried in cases of non-union, but it is to early to be sure if this treatment has anything to offer.

Eight

The shoulder girdle and arm

The shoulder girdle consists of the clavicle, the scapula and a ball and socket joint, the glenohumeral joint. The upper limb is attached to the trunk by the clavicle at the sternoclavicular joint, and by various muscles attached to the spacula posteriorly. The clavicle and the scapula are elevated by the trapezius muscle, the scapula being elevated on its medial border additionally by the levator scapulae and rhomboid muscles. The clavicle articulates with the scapula at the acromio-clavicular joint and the two bones are held together by the trapezoid and conoid ligaments which pass from the coracoid process to the undersurface of the distal end of the clavicle. The deltoid muscle takes its origin from the acromion and scapular spine and is inserted into the humerus at the deltoid tuberosity (Figs 8.1, 8.2).

Sprengel shoulder

This condition is a congenitally high scapula due to failure of the

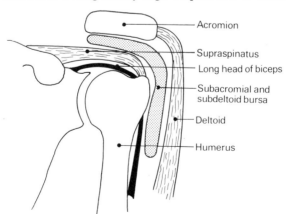

Fig. 8.1 Anatomy of the shoulder—soft tissues

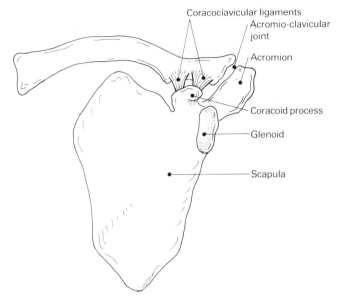

Coracociavicular ligaments

Acromio-clavicular joint

Acromion

Coracoid process

Glenoid

Scapula

Fig. 8.2 Anatomy of the shoulder—osteology

normal descent of the shoulder girdle at about 12 weeks gestation. Sometimes an abnormal bone is present extending down from the neck to the medial end of the scapula, the *omovertebral bone*. The child is brought to the surgeon because of asymmetry of the shoulders. Various osteotomies of the scapula have been described which allow the scapula to descend to a more normal position.

Fractures of the clavicle

These occur following a fall on the outstretched hand. The commonest site for the fracture is at the junction of the middle and lateral thirds of the clavicle. The traditional treatment is a figure of eight bandage, which is supposed to brace the shoulders back and thereby reduce the fracture. To achieve a long-lasting bracing of the shoulders involves the application of a very tight bandage which soon produces pressure sores; hence this method of bandaging has largely been replaced by the collar and cuff sling (Fig. 8.3). A full arm sling may be applied for the first few days to alleviate pain. These fractures usually unite without difficulty. A mass of external callus develops and remains readily palpable for several months. In Europe some centres fix this fracture internally, but this has no advantage over the closed method.

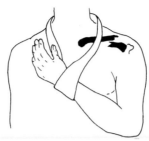

Fig. 8.3 Use of a collar and cuff sling to treat a fracture of the clavicle

Dislocation of the acromio-clavicular joint

This occurs as a result of a fall on to the point of the shoulder. The end of the clavicle can be readily seen as the acromion lies inferior. The trapezoid and conoid ligaments are ruptured, allowing the acromion to sublux then dislocate on the clavicle (Fig. 8.4). The early treatment is to apply adhesive strapping over the joint, continuing the strapping around the elbow with adequate padding over the ulnar groove on the medial side of the elbow. As soon as the swelling has resolved the pain is relieved. The subluxation frequently remains without loss of function of the shoulder, but in cases where there is loss of function the subluxation can be reduced and the position held with a Bosworth screw passed from the clavi-

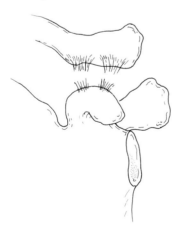

Fig. 8.4 Dislocation of the acromio-clavicular joint due to rupture of the coraco-clavicular ligament

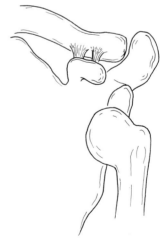

Fig. 8.5 Anterior dislocation of the shoulder

cle into the coronoid process. This is removed after 3 months, when healing of the ligaments should have occurred.

Dislocation of the shoulder (gleno-humeral joint)

Anterior dislocation is the commonest dislocation (Fig. 8.5), but the shoulder may dislocate posteriorly or inferiorly (luxatio erecta). The gleno-humeral joint consists of a very shallow cup and a large diameter ball. It is held together by the capsule of the joint, in particular the labrum glenoidale which deepens the glenoid, and the muscles of the rotator cuff. In the labrum is torn from its attachment to the rim of the glenoid, the joint is unstable. An anterior tear is common in anterior dislocation, and is called the Bankart lesion (Fig. 8.6).

The anterior dislocation is reduced under sedation or general anaesthesia by Kocher's manoeuvre, i.e. traction and external rotation, adduction then internal rotation of the humerus. A collar and cuff with a body bandage is applied to those under 40 years of age, and left for 3 weeks. For the older patient a collar and cuff is applied for 48 hours, then the shoulder is mobilised. This difference in treatment has arisen because the younger patient is able to mobilise the shoulder again after immobilisation whereas the older patient is not, and because it has been shown that recurrent dislocation occurs more frequently in the younger age group.

Recurrent dislocation always causes a nuisance and may be hazardous if it should occur when one is working at heights. Two operative procedures are available to remedy deficiencies in the capsule.

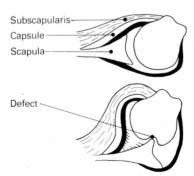

Fig. 8.6 Horizontal section of shoulder in recurrent anterior dislocation, showing stripping of the capsule anteriorly and the anterior edge of the glenoid creating a defect in the humeral head

The Putti-Platt operation tightens the muscle in front of the shoulder by reefing of the subscapularis muscle. This prevents the full range of external rotation and hence dislocation. In the second procedure, repair of the detached labrum has been described by Bankart, the capsule being re-sutured to the glenoid. The Bankart operation can also be combined with a Putti-Platt.

Dislocation of the shoulder may be associated with damage to the axillary nerve, which innervates the deltoid muscle and a small patch of skin overlying it, with damage to the brachial plexus or with damage to the axillary artery. Muscle function and peripheral pulses must be checked before any manipulative procedure is undertaken.

Rotator cuff lesions

The rotator cuff comprises of the following muscles: *supraspinatus* superiorly, *subscapularis* anteriorly and *infraspinatus* posteriorly. These muscles envelop the head of the humerus and lie beneath the subacromial arch formed by the coraco-acromial ligament, separated from it by a thin bursa, the *subacromial bursa*. Pathology in any of these structures will impede movements of the glenohumeral joint. A tear in the tendon of supraspinatus will be associated with local swelling. This causes pain when the affected part passes under the subacromial arch, the pain being experienced between 70° and 120° of abduction; this is called the Painful Arch syndrome (Fig. 8.7). A simple injection of local anaesthetic and hydrocortisone relieves the pain.

Calcific deposits in the tendon of supraspinatus will also produce this syndrome, but the deposit will readily be seen on the X-ray film. Occasionally a patient with a deposit in his rotator cuff experiences acute pain. This is *acute calcifus bursitis* and responds to removal of the deposit.

Rupture of the rotator cuff muscle either by trauma or by degenerative change results in loss of function of the shoulder and pain (Fig. 8.8). The movements of the humerus are characteristic: the shoulder hunches when abduction is attempted. Surgical repair of such tears has recently gained popularity. The important nursing precaution is to ensure that active abduction of the shoulder does not occur for at least the first 3 weeks post-surgery. A foam wedge is placed in the axilla and bandaged to the body during this time.

Frozen shoulder is a condition affecting the shoulder in older

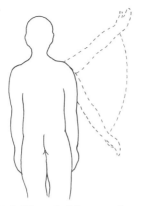

Fig. 8.7 The painful arc syndrome

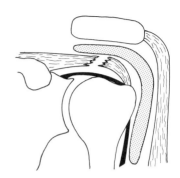

Fig. 8.8 Rotator cuff tear, in this case involving the supraspinatus

patients, for no obvious reason in most cases. It is known to accompany Sudeck's atrophy. There are three phases of this condition. The first is the freezing phase, where the shoulder is painful and progressively stiffens up until no movement at the gleno-humeral joint occurs. The second phase, the frozen phase, is painfree, but no movement occurs at the gleno-humeral joint. During the third or thawing phase, movement gradually returns. The three phases may together take up to 2 years to resolve. The precise pathology of this condition still remains to be established, but it is known that the volume of the joint space is reduced due to a thickening of the pericapsular tissues. Manipulation of the shoulder under anaesthesia does increase the range of movement, and if this is combined with a short course of steroids the improvement is likely to be maintained.

The long head of the biceps muscle passes through the shoulder joint and then descends distally through the bicipital groove. The tendon may rupture within the joint, and the only significant symptom of a rupture of the long head of the biceps is that the bulk of the muscle is noted to be more distally placed than the unaffected side. There may be some pain and weakness of elbow flexion. Inflammation of the paratenon covering the long head of the biceps causes pain related to the anterior part of the cuff which usually responds to infiltration with local anaesthetic and steroids. Repair of a ruptured long head of biceps by primary suture is rarely possible, but the proximal end of the distal segment should be attached to the bicipital groove (Speed & Boyd) or coracoid process (Gilcreest).

Common fractures of the humerus

These are as follows: fracture of the greater tuberosity, fracture through the neck of the humerus, fracture of the shaft and supracondylar fractures (Fig. 8.9–8.12). Greater tuberosity fractures are avulsion fractures caused by contraction of the supraspinatus against resistance. Fracturers through the neck occur as the result of a fall on to the upper limb. The fracture passes along the surgical neck and may be impacted. Damage to the axillary nerve should be looked for. Treatment consists of applying a collar and cuff until pain is diminished, then gentle mobilisation of the shoulder is commenced at about 3 weeks by the physiotherapist.

Fractures of the shaft are usually spiral. The radial nerve in the middle third of the humerus lies against bone as it spirals around from the posterior aspect to the anterolateral aspect of the arm, and consequently the nerve may be injured by the fracture. This would be apparent if there was wrist drop and inability to extend the fingers. Usually this is a lesion in continuity and no operative treatment is indicated. Treatment of this type of fracture is either by the application of a U-slab plaster combined with a triangular sling or by using a forearm plaster and sling, the purpose of the plaster being to weigh down the forearm and distal fragment hence correcting the alignment of the fracture. If the radial nerve has been damaged, a cock-up splint should be worn to prevent deformity until recovery has occurred.

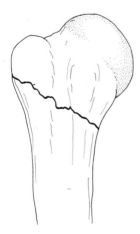

Fig. 8.9 Impacted fracture of the neck of the humerus—stable

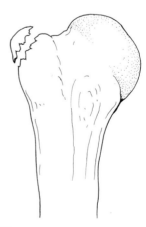

Fig. 8.10 Avulsion of the greater tuberosity—stable

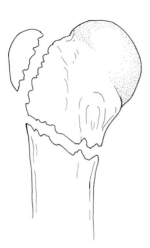 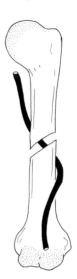

Fig. 8.11 Three-part fracture of the head of the humerus—unstable, may require internal fixation

Fig. 8.12 Fracture of the shaft of the humerus. Note course of radial nerve, which renders it likely to injury, resulting in wrist drop

Nine

Elbow, forearm and hand

Anatomy of the elbow joint

The elbow joint is a joint involving articulation between the humerus, radius and the ulna. The ulna moves in one plane with the trochlear of the humerus in a hinge like fashion. The radius has a cylindrical proximal end, the head, which is concave on the surface which articulates with the capitellum of the humerus. The head of the radius is held against the upper end of the ulna by an encircling ligament, the *annular ligament*. Hence the radius not only flexes with the ulna but rotates in the annular ligament against the upper end of the ulna. This allows the forearm to supinate and pronate (Fig. 9.1).

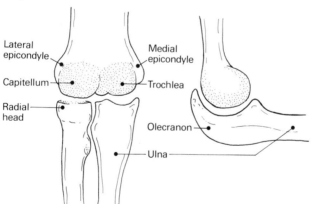

Fig. 9.1 Anatomy of the elbow joint

Traumatic conditions in childhood

Pulled elbow

This is a common injury in children under school age. The history is characteristic. The child is about to cross a road firmly held by a parent. The parent decides to cross the road but the child fails to follow, the elbow being both extended and pronated. Sudden pain is experienced and the child is brought to hospital with a suspected fracture. No fracture is found on the X-ray. The condition is a subluxation of the radial head distally out of the annular ligament, and the ligament is readily relocated by supination of the forearm with flexion. In fact the reduction usually occurs when the radiographer takes the X-ray film. No other treatment is indicated.

Supracondylar fractures of the distal humerus

This is a common fracture in children, occurring as a result of a fall on the outstretched hand. The fracture occurs at the lower end of the humerus, the distal fragment (capitellum and trochlea) being displaced posteriorly, medially, into extension with medial rotation (Fig. 9.2). Severe complications may be related to this fracture. The most important is obliteration of the blood supply to the forearm by damage to the brachial artery. Absence of the radial pulse and pain in the forearm muscles are signs of significant ischaemia. Reduction of the fracture may be sufficient to allow return of the radial pulse, but if it does not, or if pain in the deep muscles of the forearm persist, then exploration of the artery and release of the deep fascia of the forearm (fasciotomy) are required to restore the blood supply. If this is not done, ischaemia of the forearm muscles persists and they become fibrotic and cause contracture of the fingers and wrist (Volkmann's contracture).

Reduction of this fracture can usually be achieved by closed manipulation, and it can be held in a reduced position by flexing the

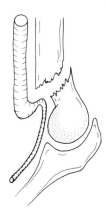

Fig. 9.2 Supracondylar fracture of the humerus. Note the damage to the brachial artery and loss of radial pulse

elbow and maintaining the position in a collar and cuff sling. Should reduction not be possible, suspending the forearm from above the bed for a few days may reduce the fracture (Dunlop traction). Internal fixation is only rarely indicated, and potentiates any tendency to produce myositis ossificans, ossification in the pericapsular haematoma caused by the injury.

Dislocated elbow

Dislocation of the elbow also occurs as a result of a fall on the outstretched hand. Occasionally it may be associated with fractures of the radial neck and epicondyles of the humerus. The dislocation is reduced under general anaesthetic, the function of the nerves of the forearm, ulna, median and radial together with the radial pulse being checked before and after reduction as they all may be damaged in this kind of injury. A collar and cuff is applied for 48 hours.

Fractures of the radial neck

These are common in children, again following a fall on the outstretched hand. Unlike the fracture of the head of radius seen in adults, there is little haemorrhage into the joint, and movements return rapidly, a sling being worn for 48 hours. The use of a plaster of Paris cast is to be avoided as this results in a stiff elbow. Physiotherapy should never be employed to increase movement, as this causes myositis ossificans.

Non-traumatic conditions

Olecranon bursitis

There is a bursa that lies between the triceps tendon and the skin at the elbow. This may be enlarged 1. as the result of leaning on the elbows as a student does during intensive study (*traumatic bursitis*); 2. due to infection (*septic bursitis*); 3. secondary to gout; and 4. in rheumatoid arthritis.

Tennis elbow

Pain around the lateral epicondyle and the common extensor origin caused by a tear in the origin of the muscles of that origin is common in tennis players, hence its name. The application of ultra-sound or injection of local anaesthetic and hydrocortisone usually remedies the condition. A similar condition of the medial epicon-dyle of the humerus and the flexor origin is found in golfers, and is termed Golfer's elbow.

Congenital abnormalities of the forearm

The Madelung deformity is caused by failure of the medial part of the lower radial epiphysis to develop. The distal end of the ulna subluxes posteriorly, the radial shaft bows laterally and the wrist joint is angulated towards the ulna. Excision of the distal end of the ulna must not be undertaken in children under the age of 12 years because of the danger of further increasing the deformity due to dysparity in the growth of the forearm bones; after 12 years the danger is minimal and it is a good procedure.

Absence of the radius causes a gross radial deviation of the wrist, which is the opposite deformity to the Madelung. In addition there may be absence of the thumb, index or middle finger. Treatment of this deformity is based on a carefully prepared assessment by phy-siotherapists and occupational therapists as well as the surgeon, and the emphasis is in the direction of increasing function.

Adult fractures

A fall on the outstretched hand may result in any of the following common injuries:

1. Fracture of the scaphoid 2. Perilunar dislocation 3. Triquetral fracture. 4. Colles fracture 5. Smith's fracture 6. Fracture of both radius and ulna 7. Monteggia fracture-dislocation 8. Galeazzi frac-ture-dislocation 9. Fracture of the head of the radius 10. Dislo-cation of the elbow joint.

Scaphoid fracture

The scaphoid bone is a link between the proximal and the distal rows of the carpus. Consequently, if the fracture is not held firmly in a plaster, union will be delayed (Fig. 9.3). Another problem with this fracture is that the nutrient arteries may enter only through the distal pole of the bone and the proximal pole is likely to become avascular. It is important, therefore, to apply the correct plaster

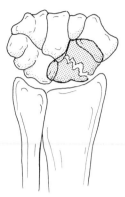

Fig. 9.3 Fracture through waist of scaphoid

with the thumb immobilised as far as the distal joint, and the plaster should remain on the forearm until union has occurred. There may be doubt as to whether or not there is a fracture of the scaphoid in the presence of tenderness in the "snuff box". In this case a plaster cast is applied and removed at 2 weeks when a further X-ray is taken. The fracture will now a more apparent. Should the fracture not unite after 3 months of immobilisation in a cast, the scaphoid should be screwed. Avascular necrosis of the proximal pole may cause pain in the wrist around the scaphoid. The only effective treatment for this is to replace the scaphoid with a silastic implant.

Perilunar dislocation

Dislocation of the carpus usually occurs around the lunate bone. The scaphoid may also be fractured. The dislocation should be reduced and a forearm plaster applied. The lunate may itself be dislocated posteriorly; this requires relocation followed by a plaster for 6 weeks.

Triquetral fractures

These are seen on the lateral X-ray of the carpus as an avulsed flake of bone on the dorsal surface representing an avulsion injury of the dorsal ligaments. A plaster is applied for 6 weeks.

Colles fracture

This is the best known fracture of the wrist (Fig. 9.4). The fracture

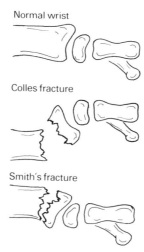

Normal wrist

Colles fracture

Smith's fracture

Fig. 9.4 Fractures of the wrist

passes across the distal end of the radius and through the ulnar styloid process. The distal radial fragment is displaced backwards (dorsally) and radially and tilted dorsally and into supination, producing the dinner-fork deformity. A colles fracture requires reduction unless the fragments are so impacted that they are stable, when the deformity may be accepted. The fracture is usually reduced under general anaesthetic, although if the patient is generally unfit a Bier's block may be used. A Colles plaster is applied which holds the fracture in the reduced position, with palmar flexion, ulnar deviation and pronation. If there is swelling a dorsal slab is applied which may be completed into a full plaster at 48 hours, although a full plaster from the beginning is more likely to hold the corrected position. The Colles plaster extends from just below the elbow as far as the metacarpophalangeal joints (knuckles). A check on the blood circulation and sensation to the fingers is essential. The median nerve occasionally becomes compressed in the carpal tunnel. It is important to elevate the forearm in a sling to reduce swelling in the first 48 hours.

Smith's fracture

This fracture is the reverse of the Colles fracture with palmar displacement of the lower end of the radius (Fig. 9.4). The fracture is reduced and held in the corrected position in a plaster, with the wrist dorsiflexed and supinated.

A variation is the Barton fracture, where the fracture involves the articular surface of the radius and the anterior margin of the bone is displaced forwards or anteriorly.

Shaft fractures of the radius and ulna

Fractures of both bones may occur in three convenient location: at the proximal, middle and distal thirds of the forearm bones. After reduction, fractures of the proximal third are immobilised in supination, the middle third fractures in neutral forearm rotation and fractures of the distal third in pronation. All require above-elbow plasters which extend to the knuckles. Damage to the three nerves in the forearm must be looked for as well as feeling for the radial and ulnar pulses.

These fractures usually unite in about 6 weeks. If reduction cannot be achieved by closed manipulation, plating may be required.

Monteggia and Galeazzi fracture-dislocations

These combine a fracture of one of the forearm bones with a dislocation of one of the radio-ulnar joints. The dislocation is easily missed but must aways be considered when only one of the forearm bones is fractured. The Monteggia is a fracture of the shaft of the ulnar with a dislocation of the superior radio-ulnar joint, whereas the Galeazzi is a fracture of the shaft of the radius with dislocation of the inferior radio-ulnar joint. The dislocation is reduced and an above-elbow plaster applied for 6 weeks (Fig. 9.5).

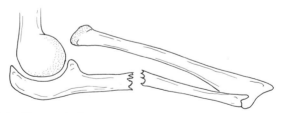

Fig. 9.5 The Monteggia fracture

Fracture of the head of the radius

This fracture is painful because there is an associated haemarthrosis of the elbow joint. Aspiration of the haemarthrosis brings relief of pain and restoration of elbow movements. A sling is required for 48 hours, after which the elbow is allowed free and the patient is encouraged to use it. Forced manipulation of the elbow either by the patient or physiotherapist must not be allowed to occur as this may lead to myositis ossificans and a permanently stiff elbow.

Severely comminuted fractures may require excision, and in some centres the radial head is replaced by a silastic implant.

Dislocation of the elbow

This is usually in a posterior direction and may be associated with a fracture of radial head, capitellum or epicondyle. Some dislocations reduce spontaneously, and the only indication of the magnitude of the injury is the soft tissue damage around the elbow. The ulnar, median and radial nerves may be damaged by stretching or rarely trapped within the joint when the dislocation is reduced. Details of nerve lesions are given in Chapter Six.

Tendon injuries

These occur as the result of either laceration by a sharp instrument or by rupture. Lacerations may be accidental, i.e. with knives, edges of tins and in industry, or they may be self-inflicted, i.e. the cut wrists of the attempted suicide. Because of the proximity of the arteries and nerves to the tendons in the forearm and hand, all three may be damaged.

Wherever possible tendons are repaired as soon as possible after the injury. However, in the past, suture of flexor tendons within

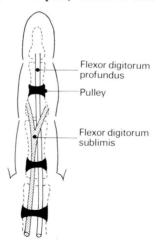

Flexor digitorum profundus

Pulley

Flexor digitorum sublimis

Fig. 9.6 Arrangement of flexor tendons in the finger

the flexor tendon sheath of the hand was not practised because adhesions developed between the profundus and sublimis (superficialis) tendons (Fig. 9.6). The flexor digitorum sublimis is a powerful flexor tendon of the proximal interphalangeal joint, whereas the flexor digitorum profundus flexes the distal interphalangeal joint. A cut sublimis tendon would have been excised in the presence of an intact profundus, and if both tendons were ruptured a graft would have been inserted to a later date. Since the advent of the operating microscope, primary repair of these tendons within the sheath has been performed with satisfactory results. Tendons in the upper limb heal in 3 weeks.

Tendon ruptures may arise because their insertion has become detached from the bone or because the tendon itself has been weakened by local disease. Common avulsions are mallet finger and the boutonnière deformity, affecting the insertion of the lateral slips of the extensor tendon into the distal phalanx of the finger and the central slip into the middle phalanx respectively. Both are treated by splintage, using the appropiate splint (Fig. 9.7).

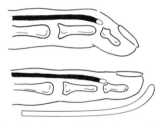

Fig. 9.7 Mallet deformity, showing reduction in a mallet splint

Rheumatoid synovitis is a common cause of ruptured tendons in those affected by the disease, while long standing ganglia may also bring about the rupture of a tendon. Rupture of the extensor tendon to a finger at the level of the wrist due to rheumatoid is known as the *Vaughan-Jackson lesion*. The ruptured tendon is repaired in the best manner possible.

Ganglia

A simple ganglion is a tense swelling containing clear gelatinous material which arises either from the joint capsule or from the tendon sheath. They commonly present on the anterior or posterior aspect of the wrist. Occasionally they rupture spontaneously. Local pressure may occur on tendons and nerves. Following formal excision surgically, ganglia have a tendency to recur.

Dupuytren's contracture

This is a condition of the palmar fascia. Nodules and bands of fibrous tissue develop in the palm and extend into the fingers (Fig. 9.8). Contractures of the metacarpal and proximal interphalangeal joints may then develop. If the contractures increase, the finger is eventually curled up in the palm. The ring and little fingers are the most commonly affected and there seems to be a positive family history of the condition in 60 per cent of those affected. Thickening of the skin over the dorsum of the proximal interphalangeal joints (knuckle pads) is present in some cases.

Treatment is indicated only if the fingers are developing contractures. Several operative techniques are in current use, but the principle is to excise the diseased palmar fascia in the affected area. The skin is also contracted, particularly in the fingers, and Z-plasties are required to achieve adequate skin closure. The operation is a partial fasciectomy. Some surgeons leave the palmar part of the incision unsutured (open palm technique) while others close the skin with Z-plasties wherever necessary. Swelling of the hand in the immediate postoperative period is avoided by elevating the hand in a roller-towel sling for 24 hours. Unfortunately, Dupuytren's contracture may recur or develop in other sites in the hand and a second partial fasciectomy may then be necessary. The feet may also be involved, but surgery is not required, as the toes do not contract.

Traumatic injuries to the fingers

Fractures of the phalanges are splinted with bridge strapping to an adjacent finger. It is important to ensure that there is no rotational deformity. Dislocation of the finger joints is associated with damage to the collateral ligaments and the volar plate. After reduction and

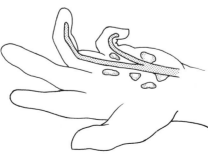

Fig. 9.8 Duypuytren's contracture. Note bands and nodules

splintage with bridge strapping for 3 weeks, these ligaments usually heal. The collateral ligaments of the thumb metacarpo-phalangeal joint require re-attachment surgically as they rarely heal satisfactorily with splintage alone.

Subungual haematoma

Crush injuries to the finger tips may give rise to a haematoma under the nail. This is usually very painful. The haematoma should be released by trephining the nail. This relieves pain and prevents subsequent nail avulsion. A paper-clip is straightened and heated on a spirit flame. The red hot tip of the clip is then gently placed on the nail over the haematoma. A small hole is burned through the nail, the haematoma is suddenly released under pressure, pain immediately subsides and the nail is preserved viable.

Sudeck's atrophy

Sudeck's atrophy may follow any injury to the upper limb, but is most commonly seen after Colles fractures. Pain and stiffness in the wrist, hand and fingers with atrophy of the skin, which becomes red and shiny, is characteristic of this condition. The bones become osteoporotic. Sometimes the shoulder also becomes stiff and painful like a frozen shoulder: this is the shoulder-hand syndrome.

The mechanism of Sudeck's atrophy condition is not understood, but it is thought to be mediated by the sympathetic nervous system. No specific treatment is known, although guanethidine blocks may be given. The limb is mobilised as much as possible. The condition is self-limiting and usually resolves within a period of not more than 3 years.

Fractures of the olecranon

These occur as a result of a fall on to the point of the elbow. The triceps tendon is inserted into the olecranon, which causes wide displacement of the fracture. The fracture requires reduction and fixation with a screw or, as is more popular today, tension-band wiring (Fig. 9.9).

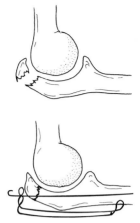

Fig. 9.9 Fracture of the olecranon, showing fixation with tension band wiring

Ten

The spine

General anatomy

The spinal column is comprised of seven cervical, twelve thoracic, five lumbar, five sacral (fused together) and four coccygeal (fused together) vertebrae. Each vertebra consists of a body anteriorly which is oval in shape. The intervertebral disc is attached to the body both superiorly and inferiorly, acting as a shock-absorber between the vertebrae. The anterior aspects of the bodies are joined throughout the length of the spine by the *anterior longitudinal ligament* and posteriorly by the *posterior longitudinal ligament* (Fig. 10.1). From the posterior aspect of the vertebral body, the pedicles arise and link it to the neural arch behind, which consists of the laminea and spinous processes. The transverse process arises at the junction of the pedicle with the lamina and projects laterally, acting as a point of attachment for muscles. Projecting superiorly from the junction of the pedicle and lamina is the superior articular facet (Fig. 10.2). This faces inwards and articulates with the in-

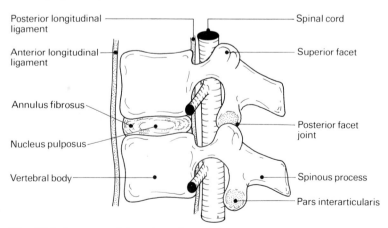

Fig. 10.1 Anatomy of the spine—lateral view

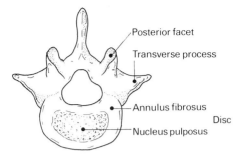

Fig. 10.2 Horizontal view of a vertebra

ferior facet of the vertebra above. Inferiorly from the junction of the pedicle and lamina is a strut of bone which extends downwards and forms the inferiorarticular facet. This faces outwards to articulate with the superior facet of the vertebra below. The strut is known as the *pars interarticilaris*. A rib articulates with each thoracic vertebra, although the twelfth is frequently only a rudimentary rib.

Affections of the spine

These may be congenital or acquired, intrinsic or extrinsic. The congenital affections may be the failure of any part of the vertebra to develop (intrinsic) or due to contractures in muscles acting on the spine (extrinsic). The acquired affections may be the result of fracturers of a part of the vertebra, infections of the vertebrae, disorders of the facetal joints, injury to the intervertebral discs or tumours; or they may be of the extrinsic variety, causing curvature of the spine either in flexion (ankylosing spondylosis) or in lateral flexion with or without rotation (scoliosis).

The cervical spine

Torticollis

This may be present at birth (congenital) or develop during childhood (acute wry neck). The head is held in lateral flexion towards one shoulder and rotated towards the other shoulder (Fig. 10.3). In the congenital type a lump may be felt in the tendon of sternomastoid muscle which is called a *sternomastoid tumour*. This represents fibrous tissue within the muscle which causes it to become contracted, producing the deformity.

It is thought that this tumour arises as the result of a difficult

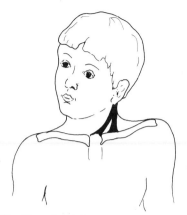

Fig. 10.3 Torticollis. Note the tight sternomastoid muscle

birth, the muscle becoming ischaemic either due to rotation of the neck or pressure on the muscle, particularly by forceps.

Early treatment is gentle manipulation of the neck to stretch the tight muscle. This is usually sufficient for the infant, but the older child requires release of the tight tendon by open operation (tenotomy). Physiotherapy should be continued following this procedure to maintain the correction obtained.

Acute wry neck occurs without a history of injury to the neck in the majority of cases. The child wakes in the morning with his head turned to one side and tilted towards the opposite side. The sternomastoid muscle is in spasm on one side. Radiographs of the cervical spine reveal no abnormality. A soft cervical collar is prescribed and after a few days the deformity subsides.

Klippel-Feil syndrome

This is also known as *brevicollis,* and is a condition where there appears to be no neck, the head resting on the shoulders. The features of the syndrome are: 1. Short or absent neck 2. Absence of or greatly reduced neck movements 3. Lowered hair-line.

Other congenital anomalies such as cleft palate, congenital heart disease and renal abnormalities, are frequently present. The only need for treatment is for decompression of the spinal cord if it becomes compressed in later life.

Atlanto-axial subluxation

In the young this is usually due to a congenital absence of part of the vertebra. The condition may be diagnosed after the neck has been X-rayed following the development of what was thought to be a wry neck. The odontoid peg fails to develop, and the axis (second cervical vertebra) subluxes posteriorly on the atlas (first cervical vertebra) and may cause pressure on the spinal cord.

In the younger adult the commonest cause of this condition is a fracture of the base of the odontoid process or rupture of the transverse ligament of the atlas. Subluxation of C1 and C2 is then possible, and the cord may be compressed (Fig. 10.4). If the compression is severe the patient dies due to respiratory arrest; if less severe he may develop a quadriplegia, or if only slight he may only have pain in his arms with altered sensation.

In the rheumatoid patient erosion of the odontoid peg or spontaneous rupture of the transverse ligament may occur, and all patients admitted to hospital for an operation who have rheumatoid must have X-rays taken of the odontoid peg to exclude this lesion.

Initial treatment of atlanto-axal subluxation requires the application of a soft cervical collar to restrict flexion and extension of the neck. Should the instability persist, posterior fusion of C1 to C2 is indicated. A figure of eight wire is looped around the neural arch of C1 and the spinous process of C2, bone graft being laid posteriorly

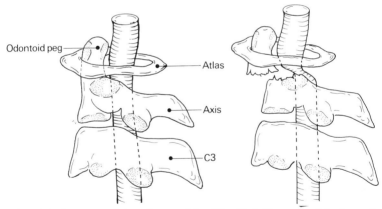

Fig. 10.4 Anatomy of the atlanto-axial joint

Fig. 10.5 Fracture of the base of the odontoid with anterior subluxion of C1 and C2 and compression of spinal cord

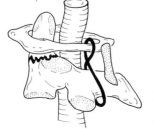

Fig. 10.6 Repair of the atlanto-axial joint by posterior bone graft with wiring

over the laminae (Fig. 10.6). A rigid polythene collar or Minerva plaster is worn for 6 weeks to allow the graft to take, then the neck is allowed free of support.

Hangman's fracture

This fracture is the result of a hyperextension fracture-dislocation of C2 on C3. A fracture occurs across the neural arch of the axis and the body of the axis is then free to flex or extend on C3.

Fracture-dislocations

All these injuries require skull traction and stabilisation if the dislocation persists and neurological signs develop. Skull traction is best applied using Crutchfield tongs (Fig. 10.7). Some centres use a halter, but this is not recommended because it is uncomfortable and produces sores under the chin. Traction is applied over a pulley.

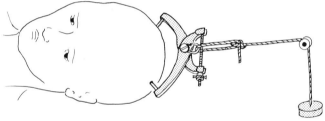

Fig. 10.7 Method of applying cervical traction

If neurological damage has occurred, a high cervical fracture may cause a quadriplegia and a low lesion a paraplegia. Meticulous care of the skin and pressure areas is vital, and a tilting bed is essential for good nursing care where nurses are not trained in turning spinal injuries. The Stake-Mandeville bed or a Stryker frame are suitable. Attention must be given to bladder function, a catheter being introduced if necessary. Suppositories are given regularly and manual removal of faeces may be necessary. The urinary catheter will be required until the period of spinal shock has passed and an autonomic bladder function is established, tapping the bladder being taught to stimulate a bladder contraction.

Stable fractures of the cervical spine

This group of fractures includes the wedge-compression fracture due to flexion, which needs no specific treatment although a collar

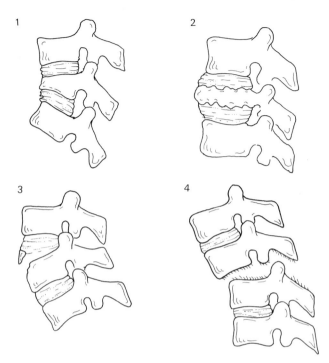

Fig. 10.8 Fractures of the spine. 1) Flexion injury causing wedging of vertebral body 2) Compression injury 3) Extension injury 4) Fracture-dislocation

may help pain, and the vertical compression injury, due to a blow on the head, in which the posterior longitudinal ligament remains intact. Despite the presence of a comminuted body fracture, the spine is stable and bed rest followed by a collar is all that is needed. Extension injuries similarly are stable in the presence of a body fracture and a collar is an adequate support (Fig. 10.8).

Ligamentous injury (whip-lash injury)

This injury is common in road traffic accidents. A person strapped in his seat sustains a head-on collision; his body is restrained by the belt but his head flexes forward at the time of the impact, then if there is no head rest to prevent it, is thrust backwards into hyperextension. No fracture occurs, but the ligaments around the posterior facet joints are torn and the articular surfaces of the joints are ground together, resulting in a stiff painful neck which may persist for several weeks.

The initial treatment is to support the spine in a collar until the pain begins to improve, then gentle mobilisation in the physiotherapy department with cervical traction may be begun.

Cervical spondylosis (cervical disc protrusions)

Cervical spondylosis is a common disorder of the cervical spine, and is the result of degeneration of a cervical spine disc leading to narrowing of the disc space, fibrosis and new bone formation across the disc space, which causes nerve-root entrapment. The symptoms are pain in the neck which radiates into one or both upper limbs and may affect the fingers. The sensation in the upper limbs may be diminished and muscle power reduced. Neck movements will be restricted.

X-rays show osteophyte formation around a diminished disc space, and oblique views may show narrowing of the intervertebral foramina through which the spinal nerves leave the spinal canal. If there is marked spasm of the neck muscles it is wise to give the patient a collar to rest the muscles and encourage the spasm to diminish. Intermittent cervical traction may also achieve this. Following this, gentle mobilisation of the neck using the Maitland technique will bring further relief of pain and increase neck movements. Abnormal neurological signs frequently respond to this regime, but if they persist, and encroachment of a nerve root foramina has been demonstrated, removal of the offending osteophyte may be necessary.

Thoraco-lumbar spine

The thoracic part of the spine gives origin to the ribs, and movement is mainly in flexion and extension with only a little rotation. Consequently it is unusual to have a disc prolapse in the thoracic spine, but infections are much more common. The lumbar spine is mobile in both flexion-extension and rotation, hence disc prolapse and posterior facet joint disorders are common.

Kyphosis

This term describes a curvature of the spine where there is increased flexion and loss of extension. In children it may be caused by Scheuermann's osteochondritis. This is a disturbance in the ossification of the ring apophysis around the superior and inferior surfaces of the vertebral body. The anterior part does not develop

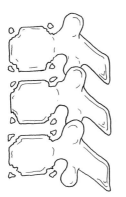

Fig. 10.9 Early Scheuermann's osteochondritis. Note the irregular apophysis

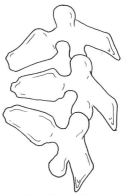

Fig. 10.10 Late Scheuermann's osteochondritis with wedging of the vertebrae causing a kyphosis

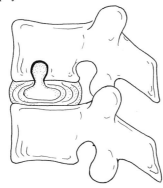

Fig. 10.11 Schmorl's node

correctly, allowing the body to become wedged and a groove to appear on the superior and inferior margins (see Fig. 10.9 & 10.10). About three thoracic vertebrae are usually involved, although up to five may be affected. Herniation of the disc into the vertebral body may also occur and this is seen as a Schmorl's node on the X-ray (see Fig. 10.11).

There is a family history in 25 per cent of cases. The kyphosis presents around puberty with pain in the back, and someone in the family notices a bad posture, i.e. bent back. The spine needs to be splinted in a Milwaukee brace or equivalent, to prevent the kyphosis increasing. This brace must be worn until there is evidence of healing of the apophysis on the X-ray.

In the elderly, where the calcium content of the bones is low due to senile osteoporosis, the vertebrae may become wedged and result in the development of kyphosis without significant trauma. Compression fractures due to flexion injuries also produce this deformity.

Ankylosing spondylosis

This is another cause of kyphosis, so much so that in the fully established, untreated case the head faces the floor and the spine is rigid throughout its length (Fig. 10.12). A full account of this condition can be found in Chapter Three.

Tuberculosis

Tuberculosis commonly affects two adjacent vertebrae in the lower thoracic spine. The pathology of the disease is discussd in detail in Chapter Four.

'I'reatment is commenced after the diagnosis is confirmed. This is done by considering the radiological appearances, by a raised ESR, a positive. Mantoux test and the histology and culture of tissue obtained from a needle biopsy of the vertebral lesion. Bed rest and anti-tuberculous drug therapy for a prolonged period are usually sufficient to allow healing to occur spontaneously. Abscesses may require to be aspirated or drained if they point under the skin, or if they compress the spinal cord and cause a paraplegia which does not respond to a full course of chemotherapy (6 weeks).

Chronic discharging tuberculosis sinus was a feature of this disease before the advent of antibiotics, but it is rarely seen today.

Some surgeons believe in a radical approach to spinal tuberculo-

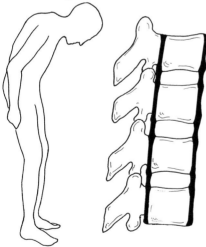

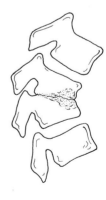

Fig. 10.12 Ankylosing spondylitis. Note calcification of the anterior longitudinal ligament forming 'bamboo spine'

Fig. 10.13 Tuberculosis of the spine

sis and excise the diseased vertebral bodies and insert bone graft struts to bridge the gap and prevent the development of kyphosis. This is not the view held by the Medical Research Council Working Party who, in 1974, advocated a conservative approach to the management of the disease.

The patient is nursed in bed, and is not allowed to get out of bed until the infection has responded to treatment. This is determined by the fact that the patient's general health has improved and that the ESR has returned to normal and the patient has remained apyrexial, with the resolution of tuberculous abscesses. When this has been achieved, the patient is gradually mobilised wearing a suitable surgical corset. Antituberculous drugs used to be given for a total of 2 years but now the length of treatment is being reduced, and in some centres is only 1 year.

Where a tuberculous lesion has produced Pott's paraplegia, or in a case which has failed to respond to a full course of antituberculous drugs with bed rest, decompression is necessary, and the longer it is delayed the poorer the prognosis. Decompression must not be attempted by approaching the vertebra from behind, as the stability of the spine depends on the integrity of the neural arch. Costotransversectomy, the anterolateral approach, is preferred to the anterior approach as fewer structures are disturbed. In this operation the posterior 5 cm of the rib and the corresponding transverse process of the affected vertebra are removed and access to the abscess in the vertebral body is achieved through the base of the transverse process (Fig. 10.14). Pus and debris are removed. The pedicles

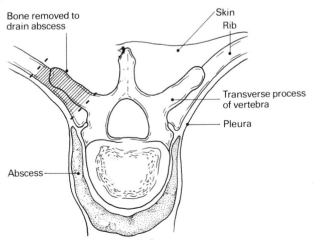

Fig. 10.14 Costotransversectomy for drainage of tuberculosis abscess in the thoracic spine

are left intact, maintaining the stability of the spine. Should a wider exposure be necessary, the anterolateral approach is used. Bone graft can be laid between the remaining healthy vertebrae to prevent the formation of a kyphos. If the spine is unstable a plaster shell is made to lay the patient in until the graft is incorporated, which may take up to 3 months.

Throughout the treatment of these patients a well-balanced diet is essential, and attention should be paid to pressure areas in view of the long time spend recumbent. If other foci of the disease occur they require attention in their own right, and particularly if there is pulmonary tuberculosis the patient requires to be isolated.

Pyogenic infections

Like osteomyelitis in any other bone of the skeleton, bacteria lodge in the vertebra producing an osteomyelitis. *Staphylococcus, Escherichia coli, Proteus, Pseudomonas* and *Salmonella* are common pathogens. The patient complains of vague pain in the back and feeling unwell. A pyroxia is present, but it is frequently low grade, and there is marked spasm in the muscles around the part of the spine affected. Radiographs reveal destruction of the vertebral body with surrounding osteoporosis and subsequent narrowing of the disc. Usually only one vertebra is involved, which distinguishes osteomyelitis from tuberculosis. The ESR will be raised and the white cell count will shown a neutrophilia. Blood cultures may grow the organism in the acute phase. The serum anti-staphylococcal or anti-streptolysin antibody titres may indicate the causal organism. An isotope bone scan shows a hot spot at the site of the infection and is useful in doubtful cases. Biopsy with a needle should provide suitable material for culture.

It is mandatory to isolate the organism so that the appropriate antibiotic can be given. The course of the antibiotic treatment should last at least 3 months. Infections in the discs do occur, but they are usually secondary to surgical procedures on the disc. As in tuberculosis, the patient requires a well balanced diet with added vitamins if necessary, and should be nursed on strict bed rest until the infection has responded to treatment, i.e. the patient feels well and the ESR has fallen to normal.

Low back pain

Pain in the low back is a very common condition, and all of us at some time in our life will experience it in some form. It is important to be aware of the possible causes of pain that is felt in the low back; they are as follows: 1. Ligamentous and muscular pain 2. Joint pain 3. Nerve root pain 4. Bone pain 5. Referred pain

Ligamentous and muscular pain

Muscles and ligaments sustain partial tears when subjected to loads that they are unaccustomed to. The muscles that extend the spine, the erector spinae muscles, are complex in their structure, and minor tears of their origins or insertions give rise to pain in the back. Similarly the ligaments around the posterior facet joints can also be affected. The patient may have been engaged in heavy work to which he is unaccustomed, and later that day the back will stiffen and become painful. Frequently a hot bath and bed rest alleviates the pain. Rarely does this type of pain persist beyond one week.

Joint pain

The posterior facet joints allow flexion, extension and rotation to occur. Should excessive rapid movements in either of these directions occur, particularly under the influence of external load, then the articular cartilage of these facet joints is damaged. This gives rise to pain at the affected level. The body's response to back pain is to increase the tension in the erector spinae muscles, which inturn increases the pressure across the facet joint and thereby further increases the pain! A vicious circle then develops of pain giving rise to muscle spasm giving rise to more pain and more spasm. Eventually all the extensor muscles throughout the length of the spine go into spasm, causing pain not only in the low back but across the shoulders and up across the head.

The important factor in the treatment of this pain is to reduce the secondary muscle spasm. This can be done by various methods; bed rest, tranquillizers, traction, heat and a hospitable environment. Exercises and physiotherapy in the acute phase only aggravate the spasm, but are of value in the late mobilisation of these patients. Frequently, mental stress and anxiety develops which requires treatment before the symptoms can disappear. Maitlands Mobilisation are ideal for treating the facet joints when the muscle spasm has diminished.

Nerve-root pain

The nerve roots, as they leave the spinal canal through the intervertebral foraminae, may be compressed by an intervertebral disc that has protruded or herniated through the annulus fibrosus ('slipped disc') or due to enlargement of the facet joints as in osteoarthritis. Within the spinal canal the nerve roots may be compressed by central herniation of the disc, tumours outside the spinal cord (extradural) and tumours arising deep to the dura, (intradural). The pain distribution in these disorders is characteristic. Pain appears not only in the back, but in the leg, and varies in its location depending on which nerve root is affected. If the 5th lumbar root is compressed the pain radiates from the low back, across the buttock, down the lateral side of the thigh and calf and across to the medial side of the foot as far as the great toe. In 1st sacral nerve-root compression the pain radiates from the buttock to the lateral or posterior aspect of the thigh, the posterior aspect of the calf and on to the lateral border of the foot as far as the little toe.

Prolapsed intervertebral disc

The intervertebral discs are formed of two parts. There is a gelatinous centre, the *nucleus pulposus*, composed of a mucoplysaccharides, collagan fibrilis and water. The water content drops with age and the disc material hardens. Surrounding the nucleus pulposus is a ring of thick fibrous tissue, the *annulus fibrousus* which is strong and not very extensible. The disc can only protrude through the annulus when it is ruptured, either as the result of major back injury or secondary to degeneration in the material of the annulus. When a protrusion occurs, the nucleus pulposus is forced through the herniation in the annulus and comes to lie either anterior to the spinal cord or its nerve roots (cauda equina) below the level of the second lumbar vertebra, or lateral to the nerve roots, compressing them as they turn to leave the canal through the intervertebral foramina (Fig. 10.15).

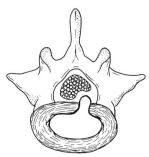

Fig. 10.15 Prolapsed intervertebral disc

The disc prolapse occurs as the result of attempting to lift an object which is too heavy with extended knees and a flexed back which causes immediate pain in the back and down the leg (sciatica). The back may appear to 'lock' in a flexed position. Coughing, sneezing or straining at stool may aggravate the symptoms, and rest on a hard surface brings relief. Disc prolapse affects adults until they reach the mid forties, after which the disc harden.

Facet encroachment and spinal stenosis

In the older patient with nerve-root compression, the posterior facet joints enlarge due to osteoarthritis and cause local pressure on adjacent nerve roots. Should the compression be such that the whole contents of the spinal canal are compressed, spinal stenosis occurs. There may be no obvious abnormalities in the limbs when the patient is examined at rest, but after exercise a tendon jerk may disappear and weakness in muscles develop. Characteristically the pain develops after walking and is relieved by rest.

Tumours

The presence of a space-occupying lesion within the spinal canal will also cause back and leg pain. Extradural tumours are the dermoid cyst, chordoma and neurofiroma, which may extend through the intervertebral foramina to become 'dumb-bell' in shape; the meningioma, intradural neurofibroma and glioma are examples of intradural tumours. Lipomata are also found within the spinal canal, but rarely cause symptoms.

Investigation of nerve root pain

A good clinical examination of the nervous system of the lower limbs is essential. This includes a sensory and motor examination, testing for tension signs, i.e. the straight leg raising test and femoral nerve stretch test, and examination of the spine for restriction in movement and the presence of sciatic scoliosis, which is a tilt of the spine to one side. A myelogram is performed if symptoms persist, and this involves the injection of a water-soluble dye, metrusimide, into the cerebrospinal fluid. A lipid-soluble fluid, myodil, used to be used, but this has to be removed from the CSF and may cause arachnoiditis (fibrosis of the arachnoid mater). Using the water-soluble fluid, a good outline of the nerves can be obtained, following them out through the foraminae (hence the alternative term *radi-*

culogram). Protruding discs are seen as an indentation in the dye column.

After a radiculogram the patient must be nursed sitting up to prevent residual dye entering the skull when there is a possibility of an epileptic fit occurring. After 24 hours of being nursed head up the patient is mobilised out of bed.

Treatment of nerve root pain (sciatica)

Bed rest is an effective method of treatment in many cases. Particularly persistent cases may need hospital admission for complete bed rest; some may need traction. After the initial acute phase of pain has passed, mobilisation of the spine by a physiotherapist, particularly using Maitland mobilisations, is valuable.

Only when all these treatments have failed is operation considered. Removal of a prolapsed disc may be performed through a small cut over the posterior aspect of the spine, approaching the disc through the gap between the laminae of adjacent vertebrae—the *fenestrectomy* operation. As much of the damaged disc material as possible is removed. With this limited approach, the spine is

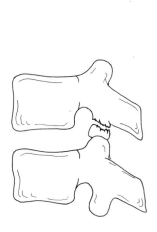

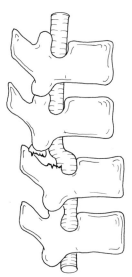

Fig. 10.16 Spondylolysis. Fracture of the pars interarticularis

Fig. 10.17 Spondyloisthesis. The fracture of the pars is now displaced, and the vertebral body slides forward

disturbed as little as possible and the patient can be mobilised early in the postoperative period. If the operation is done for spinal stenosis, a much wider exposure is required and bone pressing on the spinal nerves is removed. Postoperatively the progress is much slower. The patient first learns to roll in bed, and not until he has control of his spine is he allowed out of bed, usually well into the second week.

The patient is allowed home as soon as the wound has healed satisfactorily and control of the spinal muscles has been gained. No lifting is permitted for the first 2 months, then the patient is instructed in the correct method of lifting.

Spondylolysis and spondylolisthesis

Spondylolysis is a defect in the pars interarticularis without slip of the superior vertebra forward on the lower vertebra (Fig. 10.16). Spondylolisthesis is a defect with forward slip of the vertebra above on the one below (Fig. 10.17). The causes of the defect have been classified by Wiltse et al:

1. Dysplastic or congenital abnormalities of sacrum or L5
2. Isthmic   a. lytic—fatigue fracture
            b. elongated pars but intact
            c. acute fracture with pseudarthrosis
3. Degenerative
4. Traumatic fractures around the pars
5. Pathological due to bone disease

The defect in the pars interarticularis may be a fracture, congenital absence or congenital attenuation of the bone. If no slip has occurred, there may be some deep pain in the back, but more usually the patient is unaware of the condition. As soon as the vertebra begins to slip forwards pain is experienced. At first the pain is in the central back but sciatica can occur if the nerve roots become compressed. A surgical corset will be sufficient to relieve pain in the majority of cases, but should the pain continue or the vertebra continue to slip then an intertransverse spinal fusion is indicated. Bone graft is laid over the transverse processes of the vertebra above the slip, which is usually L4 and extended over the processes of the slipped vertebra, usually L5, down to the sacrum. The patient is mobilised as soon as control of the spinal muscles has returned, wearing a surgical corset until bony consolidation of the graft has occurred radiographically.

Scoliosis

Scoliosis is a lateral curvature of the spine. Rotation occurs with lateral bending, and if this is fixed the scoliosis is said to be structural (Fig. 10.18); if correctable then it is a non-structural curve. Scoliosis is classified as follows: 1. Idiopathic 2. Osteogenic 3. Neurogenic 4. Myogenic 5. Neurofibromatosis 6. Collagenic 7. Following thoracic surgery.

The most common is the idiopathic group. Girls are affected more commonly than boys and this type is classified according to age of onset: 1. Infantile 2. Juvenile 3. Adolescent. The cause is unknown but it is believed that there is a genetic influence, being multifactorial.

The osteogenic type is due to an abnormality in the development of the vertebra. Different patterns evolve: only half of one vertebra may develope, forming a wedge shaped body, the hemivertebra; or sometimes there is failure in the segmentation of the vertebrae causing a fusion of vertebrae. The curve are usually noticed at birth, and may or may not increased throughout growth.

The neurogenic type occurs as the result of an imbalance or absence of muscle function due to a lesion in the nerves. A paralytic curve therefore develops. Poliomyelitis, spina bifida, syringomyelia, diastematomyelia and arthrogryposis are some causes of this type. This type of curve is usually gentle.

The myogenic type may be caused by muscular dystrophy or the myopathic variety of arthrogryposis, the collagenic by disorders in

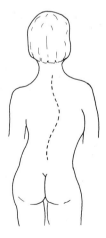

Fig. 10.18 Structural scoliosis

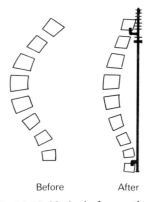

Before   After

Fig. 10.19 Method of correcting
scoliosis by postural spinal fusion
with a Harrington rod

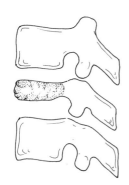

Fig. 10.20 Calvés disease—
eosinophilic granuloma

the collagen, e.g. Marfan's syndrome. Neurofibromatosis produces
a tight curve, sometimes described as a shepherd's crook.

Treatment initially involves splintage of the spine if the curve is
in excess of 20°. This is particularly important during the periods of
growth. The Milwaukee brace is the traditional method of splint-
ing, but recently, for lower curves, a polythene moulded brace (the
Boston brace) has been used and is proving both effective in supporting the spine and cosmetically acceptable, particularly to the
adolescent. Should the curve be severe and progressing, spinal fusion may be indicated. The methods of preoperative correction of
the curve are: 1. Plaster of Paris turnbuckle jacket 2. Cotrell traction 3. Halo-pelvic or halo-tibial traction.

Spinal fusion may be posterior, the correction being maintained
by Harrington rods until the bone graft has incorporated
(Fig. 10.19), or may be anterior using a Dwyer cable. Following
fusion the patient wears a holding jacket for 3 months to allow
the graft to take.

Eosinophilic granuloma

This condition was first described in the spine by Calve as a collapse of the vertebral body in a child. The disc is unaffected, which
distinguishes it from tuberculosis and infections (Fig. 10.20). Pain
is a frequent feature, but the condition is self-limiting and resolves
in about 3 months without specific treatment.

Spina bifida

Spina bifida has been recorded since early times. Hippocrates detailed several varieties. Three main types are recognised today, and all are the result of the failure of the spinal cord and vertebrae to develop correctly.

In the early days of the development of the fetus, the spinal cord is first seen as a groove on the dorsum of the fetus which is neuroectoderm. Lateral to the groove are the somites from which the vertebrae will develop. At 20 days of gestation this groove deepens and then begins to form a tube, the spinal cord. Should the process not complete the formation of a tube, the cord will remain splayed out and the next phase, the vertebra developing around the tube, will fail and spina bifida will result. Defects in the tube formation can occur at any level.

The three types of spina bifida (Fig. 10.21) are: 1. Myelomeningocele 2. Meningocele 3. Spina bifida occulta.

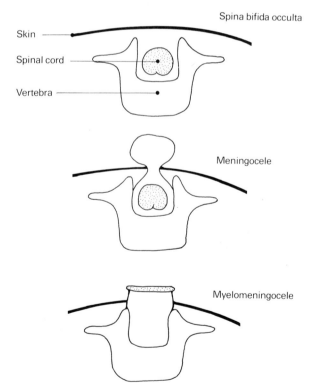

Fig. 10.21 The three types of spina bifida

Myelomeningocele

This is the most severe type. There has been a failure of spinal cord development, with the nerve roots splayed out. The pedicles, laminae and spinous process are poorly developed and do not cover the dorsum of the cord. Skin cover is absent and the cord is exposed. At birth the lesion appears as an oval red area in the centre of the defect, with a thin epithelial membrane extending outwards to the skin edge. After 48 hours the lesion becomes tense as it fills with cerebrospinal fluid. This in turn stretches what nervous tissue remains and may be associated with further loss of function in the lower limbs. Bony deformity of the spine, causing kypho-scoliosis, is present in 10 per cent, and hydrocephalus presents in 80 per cent of this group.

Meningocele

The spinal cord develops normally in this type, but the vertebral arch fails to develop around the cord. The meninges therefore protrude through the defect and present as a fluctuant swelling in the back covered with skin, which may be hairy or pigmented. There is no deformity in the lower limbs and all the muscle groups function.

Spina bifida occulta

A minor failure of development of the neural arch (commonly the spinous process and part of the lamina), without neurological abnormality, is the commonest form of this variety. It is frequently noted on an X-ray of the lumbar vertebrae as an incidental finding and is of no significance in the majority of cases, although some cases have had minor neurological changes in feet such as cavus.

Other deformities are frequently present with spina bifida, namely inguinal hernia, imperforate anus, webbing of digits, cardiac anomalies, urinary tract abnormalities.

Assessment

This is the key to the management of spina bifida. The paediatric neurosurgeon and the paediatrician as well as the orthopaedic surgeon need to be involved. The level of the defect must be established and the first line of treatment is directed at closing the skin defect and preventing infection and further neurological loss. Bladder and bowel function must be assessed. Long-term catheterisation will only precipitate urinary infection, and ileal bladder construction may be necessary.

Orthopaedic management

1. Prevention of pressure sores in areas of anaesthetic skin
2. Prevention of secondary joint contractures
3. Correction of spinal curvature where indicated
4. Decision whether the child will be able to walk with the aid of bracing or will be confined to a wheel-chair existence

Secondary deformity readily develops due to imbalance of muscles around a joint. The patterns of the deformity are related to the level of the neurological defect. Treatment with splints frequently causes pressure sores and is therefore not suitable in most cases. Surgical correction of fixed deformity is by far the most successful, releasing contracted muscles and joints if necessary. Preferable to surgical treatment are the continued efforts of an enthusiastic physiotherapist or informed parent, preventing the development of fixed deformity in the first place.

The correction of deformity is essential if bracing is to be used to assist walking. In the very severe case, deformity can be accepted if the child is going to be confined to a wheelchair.

Common operative procedures

1. Lengthening of the Achilles tendon for equinus deformity accompanied with release of the planter fascia (Steindler release).
2. Release of the hamstring muscles for fixed flexion deformity of the knee (Egger's operation or distal hamstring release).
3. Adductor tenotomy and obturator neurectomy for fixed adduction of the hip.
4. Open reduction of a dislocated hip with varus derotation osteotomy for the dislocation hip in the child who will walk.
5. Excision of kyphus and spinal fusion for severe kyphosis.
6. Correction of scoliosis and fusion where indicated.

Skilful fitting of calipers and braces together, with the use of elbow crutches enables spina bifida children many to be mobile. However it is unkind to persist in attempts to mobilise a child who clearly will not be able to stand upright, and it is far wiser to decide on a policy of wheelchair mobility earlier than later.

Eleven
The hip

The hip is a ball and socket joint, formed by the head of the femur and the acetabulum, which transmits the weight of the trunk to the lower limb. The load borne by the joint is high and therefore any disorder of this joint seriously affects one's ability to stand and walk. The hip can be dislocated, the structural anatomy distorted or the head of the femur destroyed by infection, avascular necrosis or degenerative arthritis.

Congenital dislocation of the hip

The dislocation is present from birth. Girls are affected four times more commonly than boys. The incidence is 6 per cent where neither parent has CDH and 36 per cent where one parent is affected. It is also more common in breech presentations.

Two types occur, one with joint laxity and the other with poor development of the acetabular roof (*acetabular dysplasia*). The dislocation may be diagnosed 1. at birth 2. by delayed walking; or 3. late.

Diagnosis at birth

Clicking hips are readily identified at birth and are suggestive of CDH. Affected children should be re-examined at four weeks and only about 30 per cent will still have unstable hips. This is because the other 70 per cent had lax ligaments at birth due to maternal hormones in the blood which had crossed the placenta. Ortolani's test of abducting the flexed hips elicits a click when the dislocated hip is reduced.

Clinical features

1. Assymmetry of thigh creases
2. Difficulty in feeling femoral pulse
3. Clicking hip (Ortolani's Test) and instability (Barlow's Test)

Treatment

1. Initially with double nappies, Von Rosen splint (Fig. 11.1) or Pavlik harness
2. When diagnosis confirmed, Von Rosen splint or Pavlik harness for first 3 months then Denis Browne harness until walking

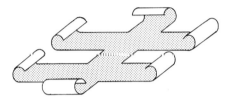

Fig. 11.1 Von Rosen splint

Diagnosis because of delay in walking

A child who fails to show signs of walking by 18 months of age may well have CDH. X-ray examination of the hips will confirm the diagnosis (Fig. 11.2).

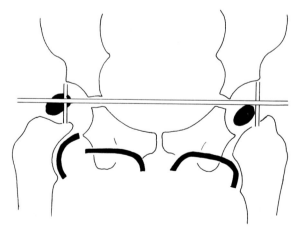

Fig. 11.2 Congenital dislocation of the hip. The abnormality in the right hip would be confirmed on X-ray

Clinical features

1. Assymmetry of creases
2. Apparently shortened leg
3. Diminished abduction in flexion of the hip
4. Telescoping of the femur.

Treatment

1. Reduction of the hip dislocation by Hoop traction
2. Open reduction if traction fails to reduce the hip
3. Initial maintenance of reduction in plaster of Paris hip spica, then in Denis Browne harness
4. The older child may require a varus external rotation osteotomy of the femur to maintain reduction

Practical details

1. Hoop traction. A large hoop is placed vertically above the hips and the legs are suspended with skin traction in 90° of hip flexion. The legs are gradually abducted by moving the traction down the hoop (see Fig. 11.3). Radiographs are taken when full abduction has been achieved to confirm that the dislocation has reduced correctly.

2. Varus external rotation osteotomy. The femur is divided in the subtrochanteric region and the distal femur is brought into varus and external rotation so that the hip is stable with the leg in neutral position when standing. A Coventry lag screw and plate are used in conjunction with a hip spica for 6 weeks.

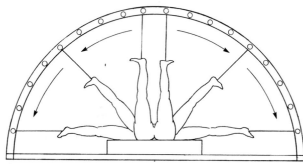

Fig. 11.3 Hoop traction

Late presentation

These children usually have both hips dislocated, the assymmetry being minimal. If only one hip is affected then the assymmetry is marked.

Clinical features

1. All features as mention previously
2. Positive Trendelenberg gait—when standing unsupported on the affected leg the pelvis dips on the opposite side

Treatment

1. Open reduction of hip with femoral osteotomy 6 weeks later
2. Reconstruction of the acetabulum if grossly deficient or creation of a shelf

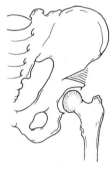

Fig. 11.4 Acetabuloplasty used to correct congenital dislocation of the hip

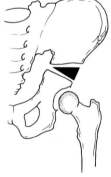

Fig. 11.5 Salter's osteotomy for congenital dislocation of the hip

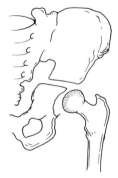

Fig. 11.6 Chiari's osteotomy in congenital dislocation of the hip

Operative details. 1. Reconstruction of acetabulum may be achieved by levering a triangular wedge of bone into the ilium above the acetabulum and making the roof more horizontal, (acetabuloplasty, Fig. 11.4) or by rotating the acetabulum (Salter's osteotomy, Fig. 11.5). 2. A shelf is obtained by dividing the pelvis just above the acetabulum and moving the acetabulum towards the midline (Chiari's osteotomy, Fig. 11.6).

Perthes disease

Legg, Calve and Perthe in 1910 described an osteochondritis of the femoral head. Previous to this all necrosis of the epiphysis was thought to be due to tuberculosis. Osteochondritis is an avascular necrosis of the head of the femur (Fig. 11.7). It is believed to occur as a result of occlusion of the blood vessels supplying the femoral capital epiphysis. These vessels pass along the neck of the femur under the capsule and any increase of pressure within the hip joint will tend to occlude the vessels. Transient synovitis, an effusion into the joint, is believed to be the main causative factor. The healing of this vascular crisis may take 4 years to complete.

Clinical features

   1. Limp
   2. Pain in the groin and knee
   3. Grossly restricted hip movements when pain is predominant
X-ray features
   1. Destruction of the femoral capital epiphysis
   2. Sclerosis
   3. Metaphyseal reaction

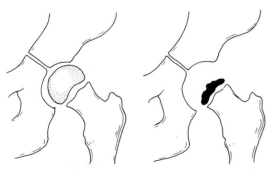

Fig. 11.7 Perthes disease (right) compared with a normal hip (left)

Catterall has grouped these changes, according to the extent in which the epiphysis is involved, into Groups I–IV. Groups I and II involve the anterior half only of the epiphysis and Groups III and IV affect more than one half.

Treatment

Treatment is only required if the femoral head is at risk. If any two of the following radiographic features are present, the head is considered to be 'at risk':

1. Lateral calcification
2. Positive Gage's sign
3. Metaphysial changes
4. Horizontal growth plane

To protect a head at risk an upper femoral osteotomy is performed to reposition the femoral head within the acetabulum, so that the affected part of the head is in contact with the acetabular surface. Group I cases are rarely at risk; some Group II cases may be and Groups III and IV frequently show signs of being at risk. Once the femoral head is contained within the acetabulum it is safe for the hip to weight-bear as soon as the osteotomy has united.

Slipped upper femoral epiphysis (adolescent coxa vara)

The upper femoral epiphysis slowly rolls posteriorly over the neck of the femur (Fig. 11.8). Because of the shape of the growth plate the epiphysis also becomes medial producing a varus deformity. Boys are much more prone to this slip than girls: the ratio is 5:1. It is believed to have a relationship to have an endocrinological aetiol-

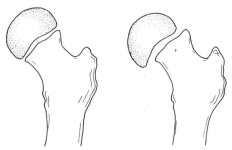

Fig. 11.8 Slipped upper femoral epiphysis (right) compared with a normal hip (left)

ogy, as those affected are either growing rapidly or are fat with delayed puberty (hypopituitarism).

Clinical Features

1. Unexplained limp
2. Pain in hip or knee
3. Fixed external rotation and lack of abduction of the hip

Radiological features

1. Loss of height of epiphysis with medial displacement on A.P. view
2. Epiphysis displaced posteriorly with metaphyseal new bone forming a spur posteriorly

Treatment

1. Minor slips are treated by passing pins across the growth plate to prevent further slip, usually three pins, such as Newman's pins (Fig. 11.9) or a threaded type (Moore's pins).
2. Severe slips require realignment either by cervical osteotomy (Dunn) or intertrochanteric osteotomy biplane (Griffiths) or triplane (Newman)

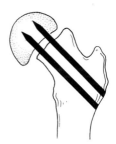

Fig. 11.9 Newman's pins used to correct slipped upper femoral epiphysis

Septic arthritis

A child with a pyrexia, general malaise and a painful hip, and unable to walk has a septic arthritis until proved otherwise.

Clinical features

1. Ill child

2. Pain in hip and/or knee
3. Restricted painful hip movements

Treatment

1. Urgent exploration of hip
2. Antibiotics after exploration for 2 to 3 months

It is very important to treat this infection early by surgery. Delay may cause the blood supply to be impaired resulting in avascular changes in addition to the infection. Isolation of the infective organism is essential to determine the appropriate antibiotic.

Tuberculous arthritis

This condition is commonest in children under 10 years, frequently with a history of contact with a person with active pulmonary tuberculosis. Rapid destruction of the whole femoral head may occur, with the formation of a cold abscess. Ultimately the hip becomes ankylosed if the infection takes its natural course.

Clinical features

1. Poor general health
2. Painful restricted hip movements
3. Possibly a cold abscess
4. Evidence of another tuberculous lesion

Treatment

1. General constitutional measures i.e. diet
2. Antituberculous therapy
3. Traction to relieve pain and spasm
4. Exploration of hip if presentation is acute or cold abscess develops
5. In advanced cases with deformity, arthrodesis of the hip

Investigations

1. Chest X-ray
2. Culture of hip fluid and blood for tubercle bacillus
3. ESR
4. Mantoux Test

Irritable hip

Transient synovitis of the hip can only be diagnosed after all other hip disease is excluded. The cause is uncertain—maybe trauma or a viral infection—but the condition is short-lived and causes no structural damage to the hip.

Clinical features

1. Unexplained painful hip, walking resisted
2. Well child

Treatment

1. Exclude other hip pathology
2. Traction until symptoms abate
3. ReX-ray hip at three months to exclude subsequent Perthe's

Shortening of the femur

True shortening of the femur may be caused by
1. Premature closure of growth plate
2. Decrease in the angle of the neck and shaft—coxa vara
3. Absence of part of the femur—proximal focal femoral deficiency
4. Unequal growth of the femora due to no apparent cause—congenital short femur

Osteoarthritis

In 50 per cent of cases of osteoarthritis there is now predispoding cause, i.e. the disease is idiopathic. The other 50 per cent have a history of hip disorder in childhood, or severe trauma in adulthood such as a traumatic dislocation of the hip. Men who are subject to increased atmospheric pressures—divers and tunnelers—and who are not decompressed correctly develop avascular necrosis of the femoral heads which subsequently become osteoarthritic.

Clinical features

1. Pain in hip, thigh or knee

2. Tenderness around joint
3. Muscle spasm
4. Adduction deformity
5. Restricted painful movements

X-ray features

1. Loss of joint space
2. Subchondral sclerosis with cysts
3. Osteophyte formation

Treatment

1. Rest, heat, traction, analgesics
2. Anti-inflammatory drugs
3. If there is severe night pain, surgery is indicated:
   a. Displacement osteotomy
   b. Joint replacement
   c. Arthrodesis
   d. Excision arthroplasty

Operative details

a. Displacement osteotomy (McMurray's) has widely been used in the recent past. The femur is divided between the greater and lesser trochanters, and the shaft is displaced medially (Fig. 11.10). The osteotomy is held with a nail-plate so that weight-bearing can be commenced postoperatively.

b. Joint replacement is now widely practised, using a high density polyethylene acetabular component and a metal femoral component. Bone cement is used to bond these components to the bone. The basic types of design for prostheses are small femoral head (Charnley), large femoral head (Mckee-Arden), medium size head (Stanmore) and the double cup (ICLH) (Fig. 11.11).

c. Arthrodesis was at one time popular. It can only be successful, however, where the opposite hip is normal and the back is mobile. The hip is fused in 30° of flexion and 30° abduction with neutral rotation. The patient walks by flexion and extension of the lumbar spine and tilting of the pelvis, hence depending on a mobile pain-free lumbar spine.

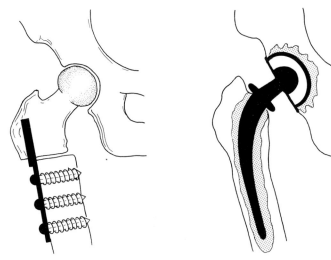

Fig. 11.10 McMurray's osteotomy in treatment of osteoarthritis

Fig. 11.11 Total hip replacement in osteoarthritis, showing the fitting of the prothesis

d. Excision arthroplasty (Girdlestone's) is used when other methods have failed. The femoral head and neck are removed, and the glutei are interposed between the acetabulum and the femur, thus forming a false joint. The hip is therefore unstable, with a positive Trendelenberg gait, but should be pain-free (Fig. 11.12).

Postoperative Nursing Care

Total hip replacement. There is a danger of the femoral component

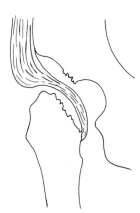

Fig. 11.12 Girdlestone excision arthroplasty

dislocating in the immediate postoperative period. Patients should be nursed with the legs abducted and externally rotated. A triangular wedge of foam is frequently used for this purpose. The hips will dislocate if the knees are allowed to touch when the hips are flexed and the feet apart. Patients are mobilised as soon as the drains are removed, being initially supervised by a physiotherapist to ensure that the hip is not adducted and internally rotated. Sitting is permitted provided the operated leg is elevated or a wedge is placed between the legs. See Chapter Fourteen for further details.

Arthrodesis. A hip spica is used to immobilise the hip while union is awaited, this may take up to six weeks in the younger patient and three months in the older patient.

Girdlestone excision arthroplasty. Skin traction is required for 6 weeks to allow the false joint to form. Mobilisation is then commenced using crutches and graduating to sticks.

Rheumatoid arthritis

The hip is less commonly affected than the distal joints. The disease has two distinct phases, the active phase and the inactive phase (see p. 25)

Clinical presentation

1. In the active phase.
   Early morning stiffness
   Painful swollen joint, skin warm
   Generalised malaise
   Other joints involved

2. In the inactive phase similar to osteoarthritis.

X-ray features

   1. Rarefaction of bone around joint ⎫
   2. Erosions in head of femur   ⎬ Active phase
   3. Loss of joint space   ⎭
   4. Osteophytes
   5. Sclerosis
   6. Cysts

Treatment

1. Active phase

   Rest, traction, analgesics
   Anti-inflammatory drugs
   Synovectomy in early cases

2. Inactive phase

   Rest, traction, analgesics, progressing to:
   Heat and gentle mobilisation
   Anti-inflammatory drugs
   Joint replacement for intractable pain

The whole patient must be treated as this is not a localised disease. Mobilisation of all affected joints should be commenced as early as possible to prevent them from becoming stiff.

Hip fractures

Two types of hip fracture are recognised: femoral neck fractures and those around the trochanters (pertrochanteric). Fractures of the femoral neck may occur at any point in the neck, but commonly they are found just distal to the femoral head. They are intracapsular, and hence the blood supply is in danger if the retinacular vessels are damaged, leading to avascular necrosis and non-union. Pertrochanteric fractures do not have this problem and readily unite, as they are extracapsular (Fig. 11.13).

Femoral neck fractures

These are seen typically in elderly ladies with osteoporotic bone who have a minor injury and are unable to walk.

Clinical features

   1. History of a fall
   2. Leg lies in 90 degrees of external rotation and is shortened

Treatment

   1. Minor displacement of the femoral head (Garden Group I &

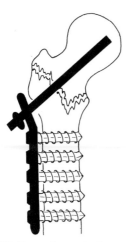

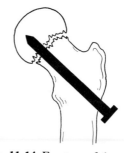

Fig. 11.14 Fracture of the neck of the femur with Garden Type 1 Smith-Peterson nail fixation

Fig. 11.13 Pertrochanteric fracture of the femur with a pin and plate fixation

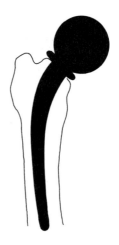

Fig. 11.15 Thompson hemiarthroplasty for Garden Type 3 and 4 fractures of the neck of the femur

II) is fixed with a Smith-Petersen Nail or with Newman Pins (Fig. 11.14).

2. Major displacement is associated with a high incidence of avascular necrosis (Garden Type III & VI) and prosthetic replacement is required, using a Thompson prosthesis with cement or an Austin Moore prosthesis without cement. Postoperatively these patients are managed similarly to those undergoing total hip replacement (Fig. 11.15).

Pertrochanteric fractures

In the young this fracture follows major trauma to the lower limb, but in the elderly tripping in the street may be sufficient to produce it.

Clinical features

1. History of a fall or trauma to the limb
2. Pain around trochanter
3. Limb a little shortened, with a slight increase in external rotation

Treatment

Internal fixation with a pin and plate (Fig. 11.13) or a sliding screw and plate (Richards or A.O. Dynamic Hip Screw).

Post-operatively all patients are mobilised partial weight-bearing as soon as a check X-ray has confirmed satisfactory fixation.

Twelve
The knee

The knee is a complex joint between the medial and lateral condyles of the femur and the condyles of the tibia. Between the lateral and medial condyles of these bones are two ligaments, the *anterior* and the *posterior cruciate ligaments*. The anterior cruciate ligament arises posteriorly in the intercondylar notch on the femur and passes forwards to be inserted into the tibia anteriorly in a fossa behind the anterior tibial eminence. The posterior cruciate passes posteriorly from the intercondylar notch to be inserted on and behind the posterior tibial eminence. The anterior cruciate prevents the tibia moving forward on the femur, and also prevents internal rotation of the tibia on the femur. The posterior cruciate prevents the tibia moving posteriorly on the femur.

Two semilunar cartilages, the *menisci*, lie between the femoral

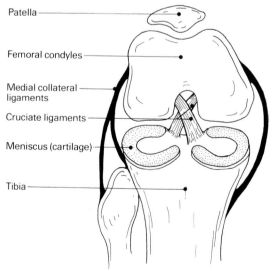

Patella

Femoral condyles

Medial collateral
ligaments

Cruciate ligaments

Meniscus (cartilage)

Tibia

Fig. 12.1 Anterior view of the right knee

and tibial cartilages, one medial and one lateral. These are composed of hyaline cartilage and function in providing nutrition to the articular cartilage of the knee joint.

The lateral supporting structures include the *lateral ligament* (which is in two layers, superficial and deep) the *biceps femoris tendon*, the *popliteus tendon* and the *tensor fascia lata*. The medial supporting structure is primarily the *medial collateral ligament*, which is a strong, wide ligament (in contrast to the lateral ligament); this is aided by the *pes anserinus* (the gracilis, sartorius and semitendinosus tendons) (Figs. 12.1 and 12.2).

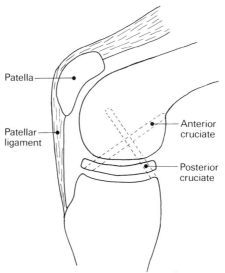

Fig. 12.2 Lateral view of the knee

Effusions in the knee

By far the commonest cause of the knee becoming swollen is injury to the knee, resulting either in the collection of a straw-coloured fluid within the knee (*traumatic effusion*) or the rupture of a blood vessel in the synovium, causing blood to collect in the knee (*traumatic haemarthrosis*). The injury may be a direct blow to the patella, or a twisting injury. Swelling of the knee that develops immediately after injury is usually due to a haemarthrosis, and swelling that develops over 24 hours is usually an effusion. Arthritis, whether degenerative or rheumatoid, may also cause an effusion to form.

Care must be exercised to exclude damage to the menisci and ligaments before proceeding to treat an effusion. A supporting bandage, either of the Robert-Jones type or wool and crepe, is applied, quadriceps exercises are organised with the physiotherapist, and after a few days the effusion will settle.

Injuries to the menisci

The menisci (semilunar cartilages) are torn when a rotatory force is applied across the knee when it is both flexed and bearing weight. The femoral condyle is ground against the underlying tibial condyle with the meniscus between the condyles.

The meniscus tears either in the vertical plane or the horizontal plane. Vertical tears split the meniscus, either detaching it from its peripheral attachment or splitting it to produce the *bucket handle tear*. Horizontal tears will produce a more localised tear, at either the anterior or posterior horn (end) of the meniscus. At the posterior horn this may become the *parrot beak tear* (Fig. 12.3).

Torn menisci may cause the knee to swell, lock in flexion or give way. Diagnosis may be confirmed by demonstrating a clunk on the side of the torn meniscus by rotating the tibia on the femur in flexion; this is McMurray's test.

Double contrast arthrography has greatly aided correct diagnosis of meniscal tears. Arthroscopy, which involves inserting a slender telescope into the knee, is becoming more widely used as a diagnostic aid, and some surgeons are developing techniques to remove torn parts of the menisci with the aid of the arthroscope. More conventional treatment is by open operation (arthrotomy), and surgeons aim to leave as much of the meniscus as possible, excising a bucket handle only and leaving a rim of meniscus. Sometimes it is not possible to leave a healthy rim of meniscus and a total menisectomy would then be performed.

The knee is supported in a Robert-Jones bandage and quadriceps exercises commenced immediately postoperatively. As soon as the

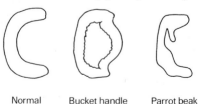

Normal   Bucket handle   Parrot beak

Fig. 12.3 Meniscal tears

patient has quadriceps control he is allowed up to walk with crutches. The bandage is removed when the sutures are removed at 2 weeks. Physiotherapy is usually required for a further 2 weeks.

Ligament injuries

Isolated tears of any one of the ligaments described above is rare. Tears frequently involve two or more ligaments. Rupture of the medial collateral ligament, the anterior cruciate ligament and the medial meniscus, as described by O'Donoghue, occurs when a valgus strain is applied to the knee with external rotation of the tibia on the femur. Disruption of these structures allows the tibia to sublux anteriorly on the femur and to rotate externally. This is *anteromedial instability*.

If this injury is correctly diagnosed at presentation, primary repair of the damaged ligaments may be possible. If this is not possible or if the instability is diagnosed late, reconstruction of the medial compartment may be undertaken.

Surgical procedures to correct medial compartment injuries

1. Repair of medial ligament by reconstructing a new ligament using part of the semitendinosus tendon (Bosworth).
2. Pes anserinus transfer (Fig. 12.4), turning up the insertion of sartorius, gracilis and semitendinosus and suturing it to the edge of the patellar tendon (Slocum).
3. Nicholas Five-in-One procedure, which consists of a medial meniscectomy, proximal advancement of the femoral attachment of the medial collateral ligament, distal and anterior advancement of the posterior capsule, suture vastus medialis to posteromedial capsule and a pes transfer as described in 2.
4. O'Donoghue's operation includes a medial meniscectomy followed by direct suture of the posteromenial capsule and ligament to bone, covering the repair with a pes anserinus transfer

In all these procedures the knee is immobilised postoperatively in a plaster of Paris cast in 30° knee flexion and internal rotation of the tibia.

Disruption of the lateral capsule, posterior capsule and anterior cruciate allows the tibia to sublux anteriorly on the femur and into internal rotation. This is called *anterolateral instability*. If the pos-

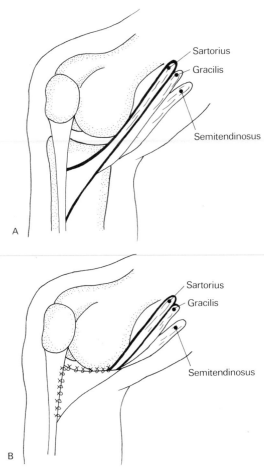

Fig. 12.4 Normal anatomy of the knee (A) contrasted with the result of a pes anserinus transfer (B)

terior cruciate is ruptured *anteroposterior instability* may result. If the knee is unstable when the patients walks, and sufficient physiotherapy has been given, then reconstruction is indicated.

Surgical procedures to correct lateral compartment injuries

Rotatory instability of the lateral compartment of the knee can be treated by reconstruction of the anterior or posterior cruciate (intra-articular procedures) or by reinforcement of the collateral ligamentous structures (extra-articular procedures).

1. Intra-articular reconstruction

Several techniques are available for replacing a ruptured cruciate ligament. The Jones procedure utilises the central portion of the patellar tendon while O'Donoghue uses iliotibial band. Lindemann uses the gracilis tendon, or the semitendinosus can be used to replace the anterior cruciate as a tenodesis.

2. Extra-articular reconstruction

These procedures have gained popularity because they are relatively uncomplicated and do not involve opening the joint. The Macintosh iliotibial band tenodesis is the best known. A strip of iliotibial band about 15 cm long is dissected from the lateral side of the knee, its distal attachment to Gerdy's tubercle being undisturbed and the strip mobilised proximally (Fig. 12.5). The strip is then fed under the lateral collateral ligament and periosteum over the lateral femoral condyle to be attached to the lateral intermuscular septum. This tenodesis resists the tibia subluxing forwards on the lateral side of the knee, and is a good method of reconstruction for antero-lateral instability due to rupture of the anterior cruciate and posterolateral capsule. Tears of the lateral meniscus must be excluded arthroscopically, and if present they require to be treated surgically.

No reliable reconstruction of the posterior cruciate has yet been devised. Carbon fibre has been used, as in the treatment of anterior cruciate ruptures, but still requires to be proven.

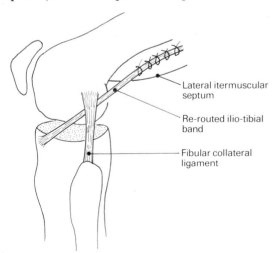

Fig. 12.5 Macintosh repair to correct instability of the lateral compartment of the knee

The patella

The patella is a sesamoid bone, somewhat triangular in shape, within the quadriceps tendon and articulating with the femoral condyles. Maximum contact occurs in flexion, and it is with the knee flexed that maximum loading occurs across the patello-femoral joint – hence symptoms are usually felt when walking upstairs or downstairs. There is an angle of 15° between the line of the quadriceps muscle and the patellar tendon due to the physiological valgus at the knee. This is known as the 'Q' angle.

Dislocation of the patella

This occurs if the 'Q' angle is greater than normal, as in genu valgum, or when the patella or lateral femoral condyle is underdeveloped. The patient will complain of acute pain in the knee followed by swelling. The knee may give way or lock. Descending or climbing stairs aggravates the symptoms.

Surgical procedures to correct dislocation of the patella:

1. Lateral patellar release
2. Medial displacement of the patellar tendon (Goldthwait, Hauser)
3. Correction of genu valgum if present

Chondromalacia patellae

This is a condition of unknown aetiology that affects adolescent knees. The cartilage of the patella softens and becomes slightly oedematous. This gives rise to pain behind the patella when flexing the knee under load as in climbing stairs. The condition is self-limiting, but recovery may take many months. In the persistent case a lateral patellar release may be helpful.

Osteochondritis dissecans

In this condition a piece of articular cartilage with its underlying subchondral bone becomes detached from the surrounding bone. The fragment may remain in place, partially detach or completely detach and move freely within the joint forming a loose body which may cause the knee to lock (Fig. 12.6). The cause of osteochondritis dissecans is hotly debated and two schools of thought exist. The

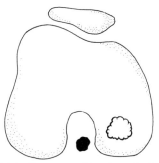

Fig. 12.6 Osteochondritis dissecans with a loose body in the intercondylar notch

modern opinion is that it is traumatic in origin, the patella being forced against the femoral condyles in full flexion. The other school believes this to be the result of avascular necrosis. The osteochondral fragments may be relocated and fixed with Smillie pins or if they have become rounded off, they may be removed from the knee joint.

Deformity of the knee

Collapse of either compartment of the knee causes the knee to become *varus* (bow leg) or *valgus* (knock knee). Both osteoarthritis and rheumatoid arthritis will cause these deformities. Initially the articular cartilage and then the subchondral bone are destroyed, causing the knee joint to angulate away from the horizontal. This causes undue stress to one side of the joint, predisposing to further destruction of the joint and giving the patient more pain.

Treatment initially involves the giving of suitable analgesics and anti-inflammatory medicines. When the deformity increases, or the pain persists, then surgery to correct the deformity is indicated. For the varus knee a high tibial osteotomy is performed and for the valgus knee a low femoral osteotomy is appropriate.

High tibial osteotomy

Two techniques are commonly used. The Brackett osteotomy is a dome-shaped cut through the tibia just above the tibial tuberosity, the tibia being realigned and a stepped staple inserted across the osteotomy to hold the position (Fig. 12.7). The closing wedge osteotomy involves the removal of a wedge of bone with its base

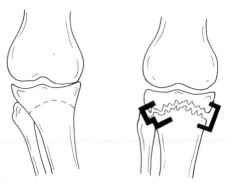

Fig. 12.7 Brackett osteotomy for genu varum

placed laterally. In both these osteotomies the leg is placed in a plaster of Paris cylinder for six weeks to allow the osteotomy to heal. The patient is then readmitted for removal of the cast and mobilisation of the knee.

Low femoral osteotomy

A wedge of bone is removed from the supracondylar region of the femur with a medially-based wedge. A blade plate or staple is inserted to hold the osteotomy and a plaster of Paris cylinder applied. The aftercare is similar to the tibial osteotomy.

Total knee replacement

This operation is reserved for those knees that do not respond to osteotomy, and particularly for those with gross ligament instability. Several prostheses are available. The hinge knee (Stanmore and Walldius Fig. 12.8) and the non-hinged constrained knee (Sheeham and Attenborough) are suitable for the severe rheumatoid or unstable knee, whereas the unconstrained polycentric (MacIntosh) and total condylar (Freeman) prostheses are suitable for the stable knee. Loosening is common with knee replacements and refinements to the prosthesis are continually being made.

Arthrodesis

At one time this was a popular method of treating severe arthritis of the knee, and for the younger patient it is still the treatment of choice today. The articular surfaces of the femoral and tibial condyles are removed with an osteotome or saw, and compression

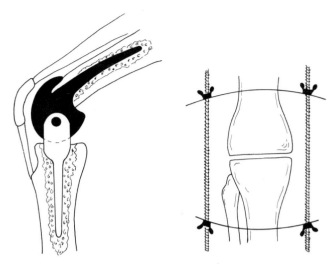

Fig. 12.8 Total knee replacement using a hinged (Stanmore and Walldius) prosthesis

Fig. 12.9 Arthrodesis of the knee using Charnley compression clamps

clamps are applied across the knee (Charnley compression arthrodesis, Fig. 12.9). A plaster of Paris cast is applied and sound union is obtained in about twelve weeks. Only one knee should be arthrodesed, as with two arthrodesed knees walking would be very difficult.

Thirteen
The foot

Congenital talipes equinovarus

This deformity, otherwise known as *club foot*, consists of a forefoot that is adducted and inverted and a hindfoot that is in adduction, inversion and equinus (Fig. 13.1). It occurs in 1/1000 births, in all races, and may be associated with other abnormalities such as mylemeningocele, arthrogryposis and congenital dislocation of the hip. Two types of club foot are readily recognised: 1. Extrinsic Type 2. Intrinsic Type.

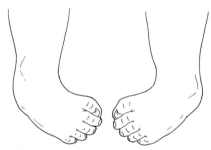

Fig. 13.1 Congenital talipus equinovarus

The extrinsic type is a mobile foot that can easily be manipulated into a neutral position, the deformity being caused by intrauterine pressure. The intrinsic type is a rigid foot, resisting manipulation. The heel is small and elevated. This type represents an abnormality in development around the ninth week of gestation. X-rays reveal that the talus is medially deviated in relation to the calcaneus.

Treatment

At birth

Passive stretching and strapping with zinc oxide, as described by Denis Browne, should be carried out on a weekly basis (Fig. 13.2).

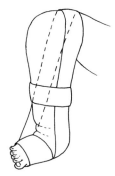

Fig. 13.2 Strapping to correct congenital talipes equinovarus

If by 6 weeks the deformity has not been corrected then surgical correction should be performed. This involves lengthening the Achilles tendon, dividing the tight tendons of tibialis posterior and flexor digitorum longus, then releasing the postero medial capsule at the subtalar joint (Fig. 13.3). A plaster of Paris cast is applied for 6 weeks after which the foot is mobilised. Night splints should be worn for the first year to prevent recurrence of the deformity (Fig. 13.4).

In childhood

Club foot presenting late or after recurrence of the deformity requires to be treated surgically as bony deformity will be established. The following procedures may be performed:

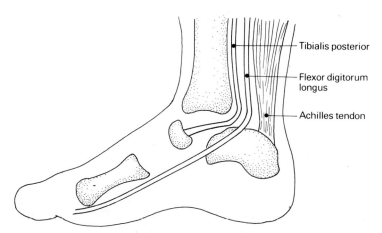

Fig. 13.3 The tendons involved in posteromedial release to correct congenital club foot

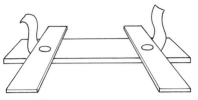

Fig. 13.4 Denis Browne splint

1. Os calcis osteotomy (Dwyer, Fig. 13.5)
2. Calcaneocuboid fusion (Dilywn Evans, Fig. 13.6)
3. Tibialis anterior tendon transfer—helps to evert the forefoot.
4. Triple arthrodesis   this is reserved for the older child where all other procedures have failed to maintain a corrected foot. It involves a fusion of the talocalcaneal, talonavicular and calcaneocuboid fusion (Fig. 13.7).

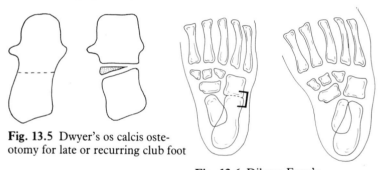

Fig. 13.5 Dwyer's os calcis osteotomy for late or recurring club foot

Fig. 13.6 Dilwyn Evan's calcaneocuboid fusion (left) compared with uncorrected congenital talipes equinovarus (right)

Subtalar joint

Talonavicular joint

Calcaneo

Fig. 13.7 Triple arthrodesis

Congenital talipes calcaneovalgus

This is the reverse deformity to congenital talipes equinovarus and is thought to be due to the position of the limb in utero. The foot is dorsiflexed and everted, the heel in valgus. Passive movement of the foot can readily bring the foot to touch the anterolateral border of the tibia. Care needs to be taken to exclude a neurological abnormality, and providing that there is no such abnormality, spontaneous correction of the deformity can be expected. The parents may be taught to stretch the foot by a physiotherapist, but certainly no splintage is necessary.

Congenital vertical talus

This is a rare condition, where the foot assumes the shape of a rocker. Hence it is described as a *rocker-bottom foot* (Fig. 13.8). The talus is vertical and the navicular subluxes dorsalwards, the head of the talus being readily palpable on the sole of the foot. It is associated with various abnormalities of the spine, and arthrogryposis. Treatment must be surgical as the deformity is rigid. Two procedures are necessary: 1. To correct the dislocation of the talonavicular dislocation 2. To allow the talus to lie more horizontal.

The first is achieved by lengthening of certain tendons—tibialis anterior, the toe extensors and the peronei—releasing the subtalar joint with a capsulotomy and reducing the dislocation holding the position with a Kirshner wire. The foot is placed in a plaster of Paris cast for three weeks, then a second operation is performed, lengthening the tendo Achillis and posterior capsulotomy of the ankle joint. A further cast is applied. Other methods of holding the talus in a more horizontal position are transferring the tendon of peroneus brevis into the neck of the talus (Osmond-Clarke) or excising the navicular (Colton) allowing more room for the talus to move into a corrected position. In the late case with severe fixed deformity, either a triple arthrodesis or excision of the talus is indicated.

Congenital tarsal coalition

Until fairly recently this condition of the foot was called peroneal

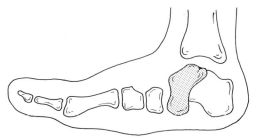

Fig. 13.8 Congenital vertical talus (rocker-bottom foot)

spastic flat foot. The foot appeared rigid with the peroneal muscles in spasm causing a valgus eversion deformity. The foot frequently was painful, the pain becoming chronic. Sometimes a trivial injury had occurred. Close scrutiny of radiographs of this condition demonstrate the presence of a bar of bone between the calcaneum and the talus or navicular. The pain arises from a pseudarthrosis. If the bar is excised, the pain is then relieved, and the spasm disappears, leaving a foot of normal configuration.

Pes planovalgus

This is the simple flat foot. The medial longitudinal arch is flattened, the heel and forefoot are everted and abducted. It is common to find this condition running in families, although an abnormality in the spine or peripheral nerves should be looked for.

Only rarely is treatment sought, and this is usually because the shoes wear unevently and the feet ache after walking. A medial arch support may be helpful in relieving pain, but it is only in the marked everted feet that surgery may help. A subtalar arthrodesis with correction of the hindfoot valgus will correct the deformity. An extra-articular arthrodesis, placing a wedge of bone in the sinus tarsi from the lateral side is an effective method (Grice) and can be used in the younger child as it does not interfer with bone growth.

Physiotherapy has been used extensively in the past for flat feet, but its value is doubtful.

Hallux valgus

This deformity is first noticed in the adult when a bunion appears. This bunion is an exostosis on the medial end of the first metatarsal, which arises in response to pressure against this part of the bone from footwear (Fig. 13.9). The bunion is therefore secondary to an underlying deformity. The metatarsal to the hallux is adducted (*metatarsus primus varus*). The proximal phalanx of the hallux subluxes laterally due to an imbalance in the muscle function at the metatarsophalangeal joint. The abductor hallucis brevis slips towards the sole (plantarwards) and no longer acts as an abductor but as a flexor, so that the adductor hallucis and the flexor hallucis brevis pull on the lateral side of the joint unopposed, causing a valgus deformity.

Treatment may be required when 1. pain arises in the first meta-

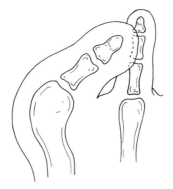

Fig. 13.9 Hallux valgus

tarsophalangeal joint due to degenerative changes in the joint 2. the deformity is such that the neighbouring toes are forced dorsalwards and lie over the hallux causing pressure problems or 3. the bunion becomes inflamed.

Treatment varies according to the age of the patient. In the adolescent the varus of the first metatarsal is most noticeable, and the hallux is best realigned by an oblique osteotomy as described by Wilson (Fig. 13.10). This allows some shortening to occur and hence restores muscle balance on the medial side as well as correcting the plane of the metatarsophalangeal joint. The patient need not stay in hospital long, a below-knee weight-bearing cast being applied and the patient encouraged to walk at 48 hours. The osteotomy heals in 6 weeks.

In the middle-aged a variety of procedures have been described: 1. Excision of the bunion (exostosis) 2. Keller's arthroplasty 3. Osteotomy—Wilson, McBride, Hohmann. Excision of the bunion alone is rarely sufficient to deal with the problem and is retained for the elderly frail patient.

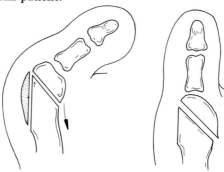

Fig. 13.10 Metatarsal osteotomy (Wilson) for hallux valgus

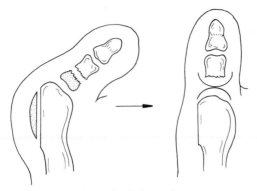

Fig. 13.11 Keller's arthroplasty for hallux valgus

Keller's arthroplasty (Fig. 13.11) has been popular since 1904. The proximal half of the proximal phalanx of the hallux is removed and the capsule on the medial side of the joint is reefed. The patient requires to remain non-weight-bearing until the wound is healed at 2 weeks, and then can be discharged home with crutches. No cast is required, although a firm wool and crepe bandage is needed for the first three weeks. As soon as the swelling has subsided, slippers then shoes can be worn.

The Wilson osteotomy has already been described (p. 149). Hohmann described a similar procedure, forming a spike for the head of the first metatarsal to fix on, positioning the head plantarwards and laterally. A cast is required for 6 weeks. The essential difference between these two osteotomies is that the Wilson relies on weight-bearing to ensure that the metatarsal head locates correctly, whereas the Hohmann relies on the bone peg.

McBride tackled the deformity by removing the powerful adductor from the proximal phalanx and re-routeing it into the metatarsal neck, correcting the alignment of the first metatarsal and hence allowing the proximal phalanx to assume its normal position. This procedure is of no value if established degenerative changes are in the joint. It is also associated with dynamic deformities occurring subsequently as this is a dynamic operation. The hallux may become varus or clawed, and sometimes a hallux rigidus develops.

In the elderly, particularly the diabetic or arteriosclerotic patient, surgery may not be indicated because of the patient's poor medical condition. Well-made and correctly-fitting surgical shoes with plastazote insoles may relieve symptoms and allow increased mobility.

Hallux rigidus

This condition of a stiff first metatarsophalangeal joint of the foot may affect the adolescent or the adult. In the adolescent pain in the great toe may be acute and recurrent. Swelling may be noted and a polyarthritis must be excluded. Radiographs appear normal initially and later the joint space become narrow with sclerosis of the epiphysis. The symptoms may best be relieved by putting a stiffener in the sole of the shoe with a rocker bar. Should the symptoms persist then arthrodesis of the joint is indicated. The adult also presents with pain, but examination usually reveals degenerative changes in the first metatarsophalangeal joint. A stiffener and rocker bar may be helpful, but arthrodesis may be required. The most satisfactory technique is a screw fusion

Claw toes

The commonest cause of claw toes is rheumatoid arthritis. Hyperextension of the metatarsophalangeal joints with flexion of the interphalangeal joints is the characteristic deformity. Subluxation of the metatarsophalangeal joints causes the metatarsal heads to become prominent on the sole. Pressure lesions occur under the metatarsal heads and over the interphalangeal joints, the feet become painful and walking is difficult. The wearing of good surgical shoes may bring symptomatic relief, but frequently operative correction is required. Fowler described a forefoot arthroplasty where the metatarsal heads and the proximal parts of the proximal phalanges are excised. Kates and Kesel described a similar arthroplasty excising only the metatarsal heads and advancing the metatarsal fat pad in the sole. The toes are maintained in the corrected position with Kirschner wires for two weeks, then the wires are removed and the patient is mobilised.

Hammer toe

This is a flexion deformity of the proximal interphalangeal joint, but the distal joint may also flex or become extended. A corn develops under the depressed metatarsal head or over the flexed joint. The most satisfactory remedy for this deformity is to excise the proximal interphalangeal joint through an eliptical incision and close the extensor tendon over the excised joint.

Morton's metatarsalgia

Pain between the third and fourth toes on weight-bearing, associated with numbness in the cleft between the toes, is due to neuroma of the lateral branch of the medial plantar nerve to that cleft. The swollen digital nerve may be excised or decompressed through the sole.

Plantar fasciitis

A painful heel may occur in rheumatoid arthritis, but also occurs as a single entity. Damage to the origin of the plantar fascia on the plantar surface of the calcaneum, in the form of a partial tear, causes severe pain at that spot when standing. An injection of local anaesthetic and hydrocortisone gives immediate relief.(Fig. 13.12). Sorbo heel pads may be useful in recurrent cases.

Osteochondritis in the foot

The head of the second metatarsal and the navicular are both sites of avascular necrosis in the foot, the first described by Freiberg (Fig. 13.13) and the second by Köhler. This condition affects adolescents and should be managed conservatively by inserting a

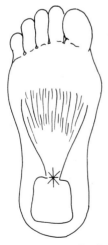

Fig. 13.12 Plantar fasciitis

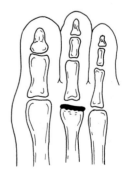

Fig. 13.13 Freiburg's osteochondritis

metatarsal bar into the shoe or appropriate insole. There is a significant incidence of arthritis in these feet in early adulthood.

Rupture of the achilles tendon

The Achilles tendon arises from the gastrocnemius muscle in the calf and is inserted into the heel (os calcis). Rupture of this tendon may occur—the patient feeling a sudden pain just above the heel and believing he has been kicked from behind. It then becomes apparent that the patient cannot stand on his toes on the affected side.

Traditionally this injury was treated in a below-knee cast with the foot in equinus for 6 weeks, and then gradually the equinus was reduced with serial casts. Most surgeons, however, now treat the rupture by suture and a cast for 6 weeks, followed by gentle mobilisation.

Fourteen

Nursing care plans

Nursing care plan for a patient undergoing major orthopaedic surgery

Patient's Problem	Aims of Care	Nursing action
Fear of hospitals, loss of privacy, operation, pain, anaesthetic	Allay fears by discussion, explanation of concepts of any operation and subsequent management	Welcome patient and introduce to other patients. Show bathroom facilities and day room, explain treatment to patient and relatives.
Lack of knowledge of type of operation, and its effects	Assist the patient's understanding	Discuss basic principles, encourage patient to talk to surgeon about details
Anxious relatives	Relieve their anxieties	Listen, be encouraging, facilitate visiting, offer help from the medical social worker
Potential problems	Provide baseline observations	Take TPR, BP, weight Test urine, record on chart
	Prevent infection	Note skin condition, shave where applicable, keep infected patients in isolation
	Prevent constipation	Give suppositories or enema or manual removal
	Prevent regurgitation of stomach contents during operation	Keep nil by mouth for 6 hours prior to operation

Patient's Problem	Aims of Care	Nursing action
	Prevent deep vein thrombosis	Use antithromboembolism stockings
	Prevent pressure sores	Pressure area care Catheterise if incontinent
	Impaired circulation	Check colour, warmth, sensation, enquire about pain
Preoperative preparation	Prepare patient for theatre	Blood investigation and cross-matching, anaesthetic assessment, shave, theatre label, name tag, anaesthetic form, premedication, check false teeth and crowns
Postoperative problems General— immediately postoperatively	Maintain airway	Mouthpiece prior to full recovery from anaesthetic Apply suction when necessary
	Maintain circulation	Regular TPR and BP estimations Check intravenous infusions
	Alleviate pain	Give intramuscular analgesic
	Wound care	Check dressings and drains for haemorrhage Maintain vacuum in drainage systems.
General care	Maintain fluid intake and output	Fluid balance chart Catheterise if incontinent or if retention of urine occurs Check intravenous infusion TRP and BP
	Respiratory function	Physio to supervise respiratory exercises
	Prevent pressure sores	Pressure area care

Patient's Problem	Aims of Care	Nursing action
	Prevention of DVT	Antithromboembolism stockings
	Bowel function	Give suppositories if constipated
	Prevent anaemia	Check haemoglobin at 48 hours
	General hygiene	Wash patient
	Good diet	Supervise patient feeding
Local care	Prevent swelling	Elevate upper limbs in roller towel Elevate lower limbs on pillows, tip end of bed
	Wound care	Leave untouched unless excessive haemorrhage or infection suspected Remove vacuum drains at 24 to 48 hours
	Prevent dislocation of implants	Follow postoperative directions given by surgeon
	Maintain mobility of neighbouring joints	Encourage movement of joints proximal and distal to area of surgery
	Wound healing	Remove sutures when directed by surgeon
	Mobilisation	Upper limb in sling Lower limb may be non-weight-bearing, partial weight-bearing or fully weight-bearing, using crutches or a frame. Patients require much encouragement to mobilise. Twice daily walking is a basic minimum and should be augmented with visits to the physiotherapy and occupational therapy departments.

Patient's Problem	Aims of Care	Nursing action
Limbs in plaster	Monitor circulation	Check for colour, swelling, warmth, sensation, pulses and enquire about pain; if continuous pain call doctor
Discharge homee	Establish mode of transport	Contact relative for transport, or if indicated arrange for hospital transport
	Supply necessary aids for the home	Occupational therapy assessment
	Out-patients follow-up	Arrange appointment and supply necessary certificates

Nursing care for a patient on traction

Preparation

Explain to the patient how the traction is to be applied. If skeletal traction is to be erected, a Steinmann or Denham pin is inserted through the upper tibia or os calcis (heel bone). This may be done under local or general anaesthesia. Skin traction can be applied using a ribbed latex loop bandaged to the limb with crepe, but this can only hold weights up to 7 lb (3.5 kg) before it slips down the leg; for more effective traction extension plaster, which is a non-stretch adhesive bandage, applied to the shaved limb suitably sprayed with Tinc. Benzoin or plastic spray, and then bandaged with crepe, is used and greater weights can be applied. Explain to the patient that the traction will help to alleviate pain as well as correcting deformity, if present.

Application of extension plaster

Shave limb and spray with Tinc. Benzoin or Op. Site. Apply extension plaster, cutting a few darts at the level of the knee so that the plaster moulds to the shape of the limb. Bandage the limb with crepe and apply traction to end of plaster (Fig. 14.1).

Setting up of traction

There are several types of traction. In simple traction the traction

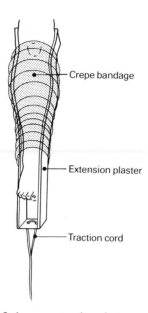

Fig. 14.1 Method of fitting an extension plaster

cord passess over a swan-neck pulley at the end of the bed from which the weights hang (Fig. 14.2). Fixed traction incorporates the use of a Thomas splint, the traction card being attached to the end of the Thomas splint (Fig. 14.3). The splint is suspended from a Balkan beam and weights attached to the end of the splint. Sliding traction is the commonest from of traction using the Thomas splint.

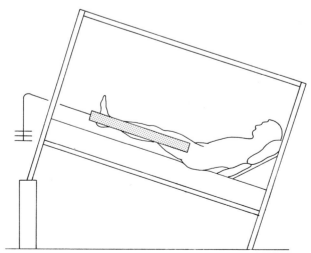

Fig. 14.2 Simple traction

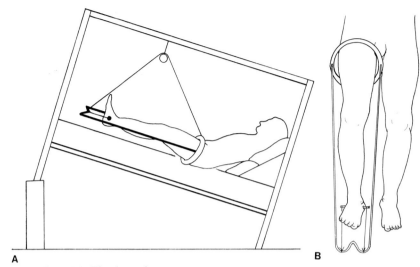

Fig. 14.3 Fixed traction

The splint is suspended as above, and the traction cord from the limb is passed over a pulley to the weight, being free of the splint (Fig. 14.4). Hamilton-Russell traction uses a sling that passes under the thigh and is suspended from a Balkan beam (Fig. 14.5). The traction cord passes from the sling to the beam above the sling and then to the foot of the bed where it passes around a pulley to reach the limb. Here it passes around another pulley attached to the extension plaster or pin and then continues to the end of the bed,

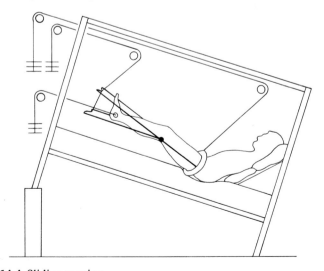

Fig. 14.4 Sliding traction

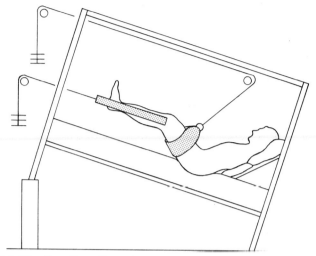

Fig. 14.5 Hamilton Russell traction

over another pulley to the weight. Traction needs constant supervision and adjustment if it is to be effective. The common peroneal nerve is vulnerable to damage at the knee by the different types of traction, and footdrop would develop if the nerve was damaged. Check the pulses in the foot.

General care of the patient on traction

Observation of the limb should be made frequently. If skin traction is being used with the latex loop (Ventfoam) the bandages should be removed twice daily, and the limb should be washed and powdered. Pressure area care should be given in all cases every 4 hours. Hygiene in the genital areas is important, preventing excoriation and rashes. Help with eating may be necessary, particularly in the early stages. Babies need to be fed slowly otherwise they will ingest air and develop wind or vomit. Adults often need bulk purgatives to prevent constipation. Assist in mobilisation of the limb on traction, and adjust the traction cords and pulleys regularly. Always pay due attention to any complaints a patient may have.

Nursing care for a patient in a plaster of Paris cast

Preparation

Reassure the patient and make him or her as comfortable as possible. If there is a freshly fractured limb protect the limb in the manner directed by the doctor. Try to maintain as much privacy as possible.

Application of the cast

Collect all the equipment, position limb correctly and apply plaster of Paris. Check that the cast is satisfactory, that the fingers and toes are not obscured and that the cast is performing the task for which it was applied.

Care of the cast

Support cast in a sling if applied to the upper limb, or on a pillow if applied to the lower limb, until the plaster has dried. Observe for cracking, loosening and dents. Any staining with blood should be carefully marked to assess further leakage. Staining of the plaster and an unpleasant odour indicates a pressure sore under the plaster cast, and it should be windowed. Check circulation by noting colour, temperature, sensation, swelling and pulses in the limb in the plaster cast. Irritation, odour and local heat indicate skin problems under the cast. If the circulation is impaired the cast should be split and gently opened a few millimetres. Weight-bearing on a traditional plaster of Paris cast should not be allowed until the plaster has dried, which usually takes 48 hours.

Care of synthetic casts

Casts made from the newer synthetic materials set more rapidly and they do not therefore require the drying period that plaster of Paris needs. Consequently weight-bearing can be commenced after a very short time, in the order of 30 minutes. Plaster of Paris moulds well to the limb when applied, unlike synthetic materials, which explains its continuing popularity. Recently described is a combination cast, using plaster of Paris reinforced by a layer of synthetic casting bandage, which combines the virtues of both materials.

Care of patient with a plaster cast on the lower limb

While the plaster is drying the patient will be keep on bed rest for all full-length leg plasters. Observation of both the patient and the plaster cast is required during this phase. Pressure areas require routine care, and the patient frequently needs repositioning. Gen-

ursing care includes supervision of good hygiene and skin care, provision of a balanced diet with aid in eating (usually because of difficult positioning), general body care such as brushing hair and assisting with shaving, avoidance of retention of urine in men and incontinence in women, attention to the bowels to avoid constipation. Mobilise on crutches or with a frame when the plaster is dry. Note any swelling of the foot and report problems to the medical staff. Should the circulation in the foot give concern at any stage, seek medical help so that the plaster cast may be split.

Instructions on discharge from hospital

Give verbal and written instruction about care of the plaster cast. Impress on the patient the need to keep the cast dry and not to poke knitting needles etc down it should the skin itch. The patient must be given immediate access to the hospital should there be any problem with the cast.

Nursing care of upper limb injuries and operations

1. Elevate in a Brook's sling (roller towel or drawer sheet)
2. Check radial pulse regularly
3. Check sensation in hand
4. Check movements of fingers
5. Check colour of skin for circulation
6. If pain occurs and not relieved by perscribed analgesics notify doctor

Nursing care following laminectomy in the lumbar spine

1. Roll from side to side 2-hourly and include supine nursing when tolerated; nurse flat
2. Check dressing for evidence of haematoma and leakage of cerebrospinal fluid
3. Pressure area care
4. Encourage fluids
5. Bed-bath until mobile
6. Mobilise when back control is obtained; this is decided by the surgeon.

7. Bed-pans are best given with pillows supporting the upper back and under thighs

8. Remove sutures between 10 and 12 days

Nursing care following total hip replacement

1. Always keep abduction wedge between legs

2. Pressure area care: keep legs below knees protected with orthoband to prevent rubbing against wedge

3. When patient is sitting in chair, always keep feet up with wedge between legs

4. Never roll patient on to side of non-operated hip as dislocation is likely. When rolling keep pillow between legs

5. Remove drains and check haemoglobin at 48 hours

6. Sutures removed between 12 and 14 days

7. Mobilise initially with frame or two sticks. When stable one stick may be sufficient, but this must be held in the hand opposite the operated hip.

8. Do not allow patient to sit in chair with the knee on the operated side flexed, as dislocation may occur

9. The patients must sleep on their backs for the first 6 weeks, then they are allowed to lie on the side of the operated hip only

Nursing care following treatment of a fractured neck of the femur with pin and plate

1. Pressure area care

2. Encourage fluids, as the patients are often elderly

3. Mobilise early, sit in chair the day after operation

4. Walk the patient as soon as possible in conjunction with the physiotherapist, provided that the check X-ray is satisfactory

5. Arrange convalescence if indicated

6. Spend time mobilising these patients as they are often reluctant to mobilise in the early post-operative period

7. Remove sutures between 12 and 14 days

Nursing care following menisectomy

1. Check circulation to foot on operated limb
2. Encourage patient to contract the quadriceps muscle by straight leg raising as soon as the effect of the anaesthetic has worn off
3. Check temperature b.d.
4. Mobilise on crutches when quadriceps control present
5. Remove sutures at 10 days

Instructions to patient with plaster cast on upper limb

1. Exercise your fingers, shoulder and elbow, if free, frequently
2. Discard sling on the third day
3. Use hand to eat and carry out normal activities
4. Keep plaster dry
5. Dress normally with plastered arm in sleeves of clothing
6. Report to hospital at once if
   Your fingers swell or become blue
   Finger movements become painful
   'Pins and needles' in hand occurs
   You feel a soreness under the plaster
   The plaster cracks
   An object lodges down the plaster

Instructions to patient with a plaster cast on the lower limb

1. Arrange for someone to take you home by car
2. Do not bear weight on the plaster for 48 hours
3. Rest plaster on pillow for first 48 hours to avoid denting the cast while the plaster is drying
4. Sleep with the plaster outside the bedclothes for the first 48 hours
5. Keep the plaster dry
6. If you are not to put weight on the plaster always use your crutches
7. When sitting prop plaster up on a soft surface to avoid swelling

8. Report to hospital at once if
   Your toes swell or become blue
   Toe movement becomes painful
   'Pins and needles' develop in the toes
   You feel a soreness under the plaster
   The plaster cracks
   An object lodges down the plaster

Further reading

General

Edmondson A.S., Crenshaw A.H. (eds) 1980 Campbell's operative orthopedics, 6th edn. C V Mosby Co, St Louis

McRae R 1981 Practical fracture treatment. Churchill Livingstone, Edinburgh

Powell, M 1981 Orthopaedic nursing and rehabilitation, 8th edn. Churchill Livingstone, Edinburgh

Roaf R, Hodkinson L 1980 Textbook of orthopaedic nursing, 3 rd edn. Blackwell Scientific Publications, Oxford

Rowe J, Oyer L 1977 Care of the orthopaedic patient. Blackwell Scientific Publications, Oxford

Sharrard W J W 1979 Paediatric orthopaedics and fractures, 2nd edn. Blackwell Scientific Publications, Oxford

Wilson J N (ed) 1982 Watson-Jones fracturers and joint injuries, 6th edn. Churchill Livingstone, Edinburgh

Chapter Fourteen

Coombs R M 1976 Supporting patients on air: an answer to pressure sores. Nursing Mirror January 29: 45–46

Fleetcroft J 1981 Combination plasters. Injury 13(2): 131

Index